THE
BLOOD PRESSURE
SOLUTION

A Comprehensive Approach to
Targeting the Underlying Causes
of Hypertension and Controlling
Your Blood Pressure *Naturally*

Second Edition

Dr. Marlene Merritt DOM, MS Nutrition

Primal Health, LP
3100 Technology Drive
Suite 200
Plano, Texas 75074
Printed in the United States of America

First Edition, 2014
Second Edition, 2017

Disclaimer

This book offers health, medical, fitness, and nutritional information *for educational purposes only.* You should not rely on this information as a substitute or a replacement for professional medical advice, diagnosis, or treatment.

If you have any concerns or questions about your health, or the health of a friend or loved one, you should always consult with a physician or other healthcare professional. Do not disregard, avoid, or delay obtaining medical or health-related advice from your healthcare professional because of something you may have read in this booklet. The use of any information provided in this booklet is solely at your own risk.

Nothing stated is intended to be, and must not be taken to be, the practice of medical, nutritional, physiological, or any type of professional care.

This information has not been evaluated by the FDA and is not intended to treat, diagnose, cure, or prevent any disease. This information is not intended as a substitute for the advice or medical care of a qualified healthcare professional and you should seek the advice of your healthcare professional before undertaking any treatment.

Primal Health, LP and its officers, directors, and trainers disclaim any warranties (express or implied), of merchantability, or fitness for any particular purpose, and shall in no event be held liable to any party for any direct, indirect, punitive, special, incidental or other consequential damages arising directly or indirectly from any use of this material, which is provided "as is", and without warranties.

Editor's Preface

It has been two years since we here at Primal Health published Dr. Marlene Merritt's influential guide to lowering your blood pressure naturally. During this time, we have heard back from thousands of interested readers who still had questions and concerns that they wanted to hear more about. With that in mind, we are excited to be releasing this brand new edition that continues to address a natural approach to reducing blood pressure based on the most up-to-date scientific research and developments.

In our newest publication, you will find current, relevant information regarding cholesterol, weight loss, and nutrition. We have included all new discussions about the importance of including dietary supplements into your daily routine, and we have taken a closer look at some of the harms of prescription medication. Additionally, we have taken the time to analyze the benefits and risks of using smart phone apps to help you track your health. And this is only the beginning of the new material you will find here.

Indeed, this is more than just a new edition of Dr. Marlene's important work, it is a renewal of Primal Health's commitment to helping people across the world navigate their way through the minefield of contrasting and often contradictory information about health and wellness. By providing simple solutions, with cleverness, wit, and most of all, her sensitivity to the real struggle of dealing with high blood pressure, Dr. Merritt's books have helped hundreds of thousands of people live happier, healthier, and longer lives.

We are happy to bring to you this new edition of her work and to meet you on your journey toward great health. You have made the right choice!

Dedication

When I was 19 and in college, I was diagnosed with a heart condition that had damaged one of my valves. I was on the cycling team but had to quit because I had chest pain and shortness of breath just walking up stairs, never mind riding my bike in a race.

I suffered with this condition for another 15 years.

But when I was 35, I went to go see a different type of doctor —one who was interested in nutrition. He told me that I had chest pain and shortness of breath because my heart tissue was malnourished. He gave me supplements that supported my heart, and also taught me what I could do to help my heart. A year later, I rode my bicycle across the United States in 26 days, averaging 135 miles per day. While it was the hardest thing I've ever done, it never would have been possible if someone hadn't started talking to me about what else I could do—besides take medication that wasn't really helping. Nutrition changed my life, and I'm hoping it will change yours, too.

So, I am dedicating this book to everyone who wants some choices in their healthcare, and to my Mom, who was the first person who taught me to think outside of the box.

Marlene Merritt

Contents

INTRODUCTION

A Silent Epidemic

On behalf of the entire Primal Health team, I want to thank you for purchasing the Blood Pressure Solution!

This guide is more than just a collection of commonly found advice; it's a system that works to tackle high blood pressure holistically and from many different angles. Instead of targeting the symptoms, which is what medications do, we attack the underlying causes of high blood pressure. This method creates a synergistic effect that will dramatically elevate your health, and in turn, reduce your blood pressure to normal levels.

Let me be clear: I am not suggesting that you avoid your doctor! What I am suggesting is that you consider, just maybe, that the fuel you put into your body has a direct impact on how your body functions. The solutions I offer aren't weird or controversial, they just remove the things that increase your blood pressure and incorporate the things that naturally lower it. It's pretty simple, really.

Now, I don't know if you bought this book yourself, or if you got this from a parent or significant other giving you a not-so-subtle hint. Either way, we are going to begin with the assumption that you have either been diagnosed or feel pretty confident that you have prehypertension or hypertension (high blood pressure).

Unfortunately, most people never find out until it's too late.

Silent Killer

Before I begin teaching you how to naturally lower your blood pressure, I want you to fully realize just how serious hypertension really is.

High blood pressure has been called the 'silent killer' because much of the damage it causes does not immediately present any noticeable signs such as pain or discomfort. Instead, it works silently to undermine your health with devastating consequences.

So let's start with some facts:

Did you know that high blood pressure is indicated as either the primary or contributing cause of death for over 1,000 deaths per day in the United States alone?[1] It's the leading cause of strokes and a major cause of heart attacks. About 69% of people who have a first heart attack, 77% who have a first stroke, and 74% who have congestive heart failure also have high blood pressure.[2]

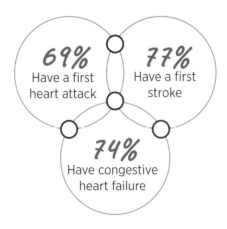

High Blood Pressure Related Health Issues

69% Have a first heart attack

77% Have a first stroke

74% Have congestive heart failure

The Blood Pressure Solution

In the United States, over 31% of the adult population has high blood pressure. That's almost one in three adults! Another 30% of the U.S. population suffers from prehypertension, which means that their elevated blood pressure readings are not yet high enough to be causing serious damage, but without immediate dietary and lifestyle changes, they'll be getting there soon.

All told, around 160 million U.S. adults are suffering with a condition that, when uncontrolled, can lead them to having a stroke, heart attack, kidney damage, and even brain damage.

As you can see from these statistics, high blood pressure is not only a silent killer, but it has also become a silent epidemic.

CHAPTER 1

Understanding Blood Pressure

Before you can fix something, you have to understand how it works. Blood pressure doesn't have to be a mystery—in fact, it's really more of a mechanical problem than anything else. So to start, I'll explain what blood pressure is, and later, I'll show you the seven levers that we can manipulate in order to naturally control it.

What Is Blood Pressure?

With all the numbers you have to keep track of, you may be a bit confused about this one and what exactly those numbers represent. Quite literally, the numbers associated with your blood pressure readings indicate the exact amount of pressure being exerted on the walls of your blood vessels as your blood flows through your body at a given time.[1]

Your blood vessels are basically a set of interconnected tubes: arteries, which carry oxygen-rich blood from the heart to your organs and cells; and veins, which carry your blood back to your heart again.[2] (There. Who knew your high school bio class would be so useful?)

The Blood Pressure Solution

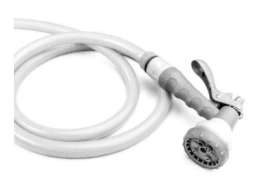

When we talk about blood pressure, we are referring to the amount of force created as your blood is rushing through your arteries. It's just like water running through a garden hose. The amount of force created by the water as it flows through the hose determines whether or not the hose stays open.

If your blood pressure is too low, blood can't be transported properly to all the cells of your body. If it's too high, it damages those vessels and can make them burst.[3] This is why it's important to keep your blood pressure within the normal range to maintain optimum health.

What Do The Numbers Mean?

When your heart is at rest, your blood pressure is lower. This is the diastolic pressure, represented by the bottom number of your blood pressure reading. Ideally, you want this number to be close to 80.

As your heart begins actively pumping, it exerts more pressure on the walls of your blood vessels. That's where we get the higher number, called systolic pressure. You want this to be close to 120.

Blood Pressure Management Chart

■ Normal   ■ Pre Hypertension   ■ Hypertension

Blood Pressure Category	Blood Pressure Reading in mmHg		
	Minimum	Maximum	
High Blood Pressure - stage 4 (Hypertension - stage 4)	Above 210 / Above 120		**Hypersensitive Crisis**
High Blood Pressure - stage 3 (Hypertension - stage 3)	180 / 110	210 / 120	
High Blood Pressure - stage 2 (Hypertension - stage 2)	160 / 100	179 / 109	
High Blood Pressure - stage 1 (Hypertension - stage 1)	140 / 90	159 / 99	
Pre-High Blood Pressure (Pre-Hypertension)	130 / 85	139 / 89	
High Normal Blood Pressure	121 / 81	129 / 84	**Normal Blood Pressure**
Normal Blood Pressure (Ideal Blood Pressure)	100 / 65	120 / 80	
Low Normal Blood Pressure	90 / 60	99 / 64	
Low Blood Pressure (Moderate Hypotension)	70 / 40	89 / 59	
Too Low Blood Pressure (Severe Hypotension)	50 / 35	69 / 39	**Dangerously Low Blood Pressure**
Extremely Low Blood Pressure (Extremely Severe Hypotension)	Below 50 / Below 35		

Again, these numbers are the actual measurements of pressure being applied to the artery walls. Having high blood pressure one time isn't a big problem. Stress, infections, and activity can cause changes in blood pressure. But if you consistently take readings when you're at rest, and they're consistently high, then you need to pay attention.

The bottom number is the one you need to pay the most attention to. It's not as likely to fluctuate with other changes in the body. When the bottom number is high, you're more at risk for problems.

Cholesterol and Blood Pressure

One of the main connections medicine has made in the heart disease puzzle over the last century is the one between blood pressure and cholesterol. And that connection is a strong one—though it's not necessarily what people think it is.

So to start, let's talk about what cholesterol actually is. Cholesterol is a waxy substance produced by all animals. It's in every cell in your body, and it's a precursor to a huge number of hormones, vitamins, and digestive acids. So it's obviously a pretty critical thing for us to have for cell membranes. It's measured in milligrams per deciliter (mg/dL), so when a doctor shows you your cholesterol numbers, you're literally seeing what represents the weight of the cholesterol that is contained in the amount of blood in your body.

The American Heart Association's recommendations for two different kinds of cholesterol can vary depending on an individual's race, sex, and medical history, but the National Heart, Lung, and Blood Institute has laid out these general guidelines:

Total Cholesterol Level	Category
Less than 200mg/dL	Desirable
200-239mg/dL	Borderline high
240mg/dL and above	High
LDL Cholesterol Level	**LDL Cholesterol Category**
Less than 100mg/dL	Optimal
100-129mg/dL	Near optimal/above optimal
130-159mg/dL	Borderline high
160-189 mg/dL	High
190 mg/dL and above	Very High
HDL Cholesterol Level	**HDL Cholesterol Category**
Less than 40 mg/dL	A major risk factor for heart disease
40-59 mg/dL	The higher, the better
60 mg/dL and higher	Considered protective against heart disease

The different types of cholesterol do very different things. HDL (high density lipoprotein) is commonly called "good" cholesterol, since it transports cholesterol to the liver where it's recycled and used for other essential processes in your body. LDL (low-density lipoprotein), meanwhile, is commonly called "bad" cholesterol, because in the 1980s, scientists noticed that people with high blood pressure and heart disease also had high rates of LDL, and from there they concluded that high LDL was bad.

But the connection is actually a bit more complicated than that. It turns out there are two kinds of LDL—commonly referred to as "pattern A" (or "large, fluffy"), and "pattern B" (or "small, dense") LDL. Going back to our garden hose analogy, it's like limescale buildup inside the hose. After a while, it'll narrow the passageway, reduce the hose's flexibility, and create potential blockages, all of which increases the pressure inside the hose. In our blood vessels, we call this atherosclerosis.

The large-fluffy (pattern A) LDL, however, doesn't do this. It just passes through, completely innocuously. This is important, because there are a lot of foods (e.g., saturated fat) that raise HDL and large-fluffy LDL—and these are foods that we started cutting out of our diets in the 1980s, with terrible results.

The American Heart Association still recommends keeping the combined LDL numbers low, but scientists are starting to recognize a lack of evidence showing that lowering LDL generally doesn't actually provide any benefits, and it could actually cause harm.[4]

It's also important to note that *blood cholesterol and dietary cholesterol is not the same thing.* You see, all animals produce cholesterol, therefore any animal products that we eat have cholesterol in them—including meat, eggs, and dairy. But the cholesterol in the food does not flow directly into the bloodstream, and in fact, our bodies' worst enemy is something that doesn't have cholesterol in it at all—sugar. More on that in Chapter 3.

Competing Advice About High Blood Pressure

There is a lot of competing advice out there about the best way to lower your blood pressure. Just go to your local library and search the shelves. You could also do a simple internet search for the answer, and you will find years worth of conflicting information that is often either incomplete or just completely wrong.

The three most commonly discussed issues you will find related to lowering blood pressure are reducing salt intake, reducing your weight, and increasing your activity. In fact, if you look at the American Heart Association's website, you will see that these first three pieces of advice are included in the list of suggestions for preventing and treating high blood pressure. I will discuss each of these in greater detail in later chapters, but as a preview of what will come, let's clear up some misconceptions right now.

Reducing salt intake is definitely important, but it is not likely to occur where you think. Adding salt (in moderation) to your food while cooking or at the table is fine—it's the salt that comes from processed foods that you should worry about. In reality, reducing your carbohydrate and sugar intake is far more important than reducing salt intake.

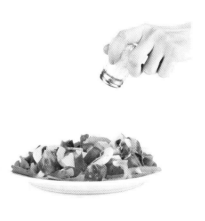

Losing weight is also important—for everybody. Not only does excess weight make us more likely to have problems with high blood pressure, but it is also associated with a world of other problems, including diabetes and even dementia. More than likely, you've heard that the best way to lose weight is by eating low-fat foods and by counting your calories, but I'll show you later why this old way of thinking is much less effective than you'd think.

Finally, exercise can definitely help stretch out your arteries and get your blood flowing more freely and easily, and maintaining a consistent exercise regimen is certainly important. However, this doesn't mean hitting the gym every day or overwhelming yourself with complicated routines for an hour a day. Doing small bursts of exercise in short periods of time, and generally being more energetic in your activities of daily living, have the potential to do so much more.

But before we get to all of that, we first have to understand how blood pressure can change, and what role we play in changing it.

How Can We Change Our Blood Pressure?

Let's return to our garden hose example, and let's also think about what factors could have an impact on the pressure inside the hose as water is flowing through it. This will give us a clue as to how we plan to control your blood pressure.

A garden hose is simply a flexible tube, much like a blood vessel. In our example, let's assume we have a pump on the end of the garden hose that is going to rhythmically push the water through the hose, just like your heart pushes blood through your blood vessels.

Now, what can we change to impact the amount of pressure being put on the interior walls of the garden hose?

- The amount of water flowing inside the hose (the more water that's flowing, the higher the pressure);

- The viscosity of the water (how freely it flows due to its thickness or thinness—if we try to pump maple syrup through that hose, the pressure will be greater);

- The force of the pump pushing the water through the hose;

- The rate at which the pump cycles and pushes water through the hose;

- The flexibility of the hose walls to expand and create more interior space inside the hose;

- The external pressure being applied to the outside walls of the hose; and

- Any blockages or deposits inside the hose that reduce its interior space.

Believe it or not, these are the same seven variables that we can manipulate through our diet and other lifestyle changes to affect how blood flows through our arteries and veins:

The Seven Blood Pressure Levers:

- The amount of blood inside our blood vessels;
- The viscosity of our blood (how thin or thick it is);
- The strength of our heart;
- The rate of our heartbeat;
- The flexibility, or ability for our blood vessels to relax and be less tense;
- External pressure applied on our blood vessels
- Blockages within or blood vessels

These seven variables are keys to knowing how to lower your blood pressure. They're actually the same variables that modern medicine focuses on with its medicines, and they're the same ones that we're going to impact with diet and other lifestyle changes.

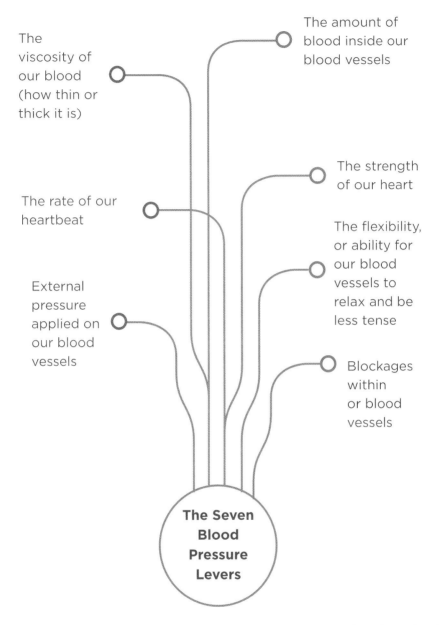

The viscosity of our blood (how thin or thick it is)

The amount of blood inside our blood vessels

The strength of our heart

The rate of our heartbeat

The flexibility, or ability for our blood vessels to relax and be less tense

External pressure applied on our blood vessels

Blockages within or blood vessels

The Seven Blood Pressure Levers

We'll cover more on all of that later. First, let's look at how high blood pressure damages our vessels, and other associated problems.

CHAPTER 2

The Hidden Dangers of High Blood Pressure

Perhaps the most insidious thing about high blood pressure is that it presents almost no symptoms that you can readily identify. Instead, it silently undermines your health from the inside out, eventually leading to a stunning array of devastating and life-threatening conditions, many of which you might find surprising.

Breaking Down Blood Vessels

High blood pressure can cause serious destruction of the vessels that move the blood throughout your body. Constantly high pressure hardens the cells on the inside of your blood vessels—in particular the arteries, which are coming straight from the heart and are therefore under much more pressure than the veins.

Now, you might think that harder is stronger, but it's actually just the opposite. The tissue of the blood vessels needs to be elastic, so that it can stretch when pressure increases, and then go back to its original shape when pressure decreases. When arteries become hard, they lose the ability to expand and contract. This absence of elasticity leads to all kinds of problems.

The Blood Pressure Solution

Aneurysms are weak areas of arterial walls that balloon out. Like a balloon, the walls become thinner as it increases in size, and the pressure becomes greater until it pops. When this happens in your brain, we call that a stroke—a potentially deadly event in which part of your brain is deprived of oxygen and nutrients, causing brain cell death.

Another impact from high blood pressure is damage to the inner lining of your blood vessels, called your endothelial lining. Alarming research is beginning to indicate that having a damaged endothelial lining can actually CAUSE hypertension, diabetes, and a whole swath of other damaging health issues.

But when it comes to harming the endothelial lining, high blood pressure is not the only offender—high blood sugar, sleep apnea, smoking, and even nutritional deficiencies can also play a major role.

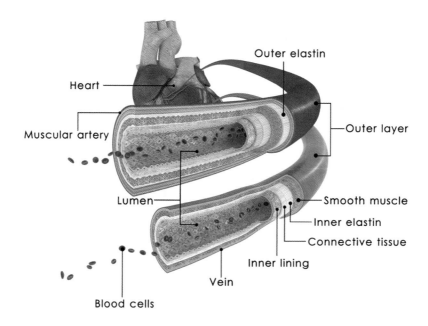

Meanwhile, inflammation can lead to arterial blockages, which in turn reduces the amount of nutrients and oxygen being delivered to your cells. Things get really serious when these blockages prevent the heart from getting enough oxygen—a heart attack occurs, and the tissue actually dies. And if the clot forms in the arteries leading to the brain, the same thing happens there, leading to another kind of stroke.

Then there's the dangerous combination of high blood pressure and unstable plaque. Everyone has some plaque (even kids!), but as we age and eat badly, that plaque can become unstable.[1] High blood pressure can cause pieces to break off, which then lodge someplace where it blocks blood flow—like your kidneys, your heart (yep, there's another heart attack), or your brain (and there's another stroke).[2]

If this all sounds pretty scary, it should. Heart disease and stroke are the number one killers of both men and women, higher than any cancers or other illnesses. So you can see how these individual conditions can suddenly become an interrelated cycle of destruction.

This isn't something to be taken lightly.

Hurting Your Heart

Believe it or not, when you have hypertension your heart has even more to worry about than just a heart attack. When your heart is constantly under arterial high blood pressure, it has to work harder. This extra effort simply wears your heart out. Your heart is then not able to pump nutrients and gases to the tissues, which affects all systems of the body.

So even if you don't have a heart attack, you can still suffer from heart failure. And if you *have* had a heart attack, this progression can happen even faster.

You can also have problems specifically affecting the coronary arteries (the tubes that supply blood to your heart). If they become hardened or blocked, not only is there the additional risk of heart attack, but also your heart performs at a lower rate and can give you an irregular heartbeat or chest pain.

High blood pressure can also enlarge one side of your heart. Normally your heart is about the size of your fist, but when one side becomes larger, it performs less efficiently.

Killing Your Kidneys

Many people don't know that the kidneys help to regulate your blood pressure by decreasing or increasing the fluid in your blood.

Within your kidneys are millions of tiny blood vessels that become damaged when they're exposed to constant high pressure—the same way all the other blood vessels get damaged. This leads to scarring, which reduces your kidneys' ability to do their job of filtering blood. That leads to kidney disease: the more scarring your kidneys have, the less able they are to filter that waste, and the worse things get.

What do you think happens if the arteries to the kidneys become blocked? Well, then they can't filter the waste, and we call that kidney failure. When your kidneys fail, you may have a buildup of toxins, as well as swelling due to an increased amount of bodily fluids. Over time you may require dialysis, a procedure that involves rerouting your blood through an external machine that filters the blood and sends it back to the body.

Ultimately, you may need a kidney transplant. However, the list for a transplant is very long, and the poorer your overall health is, the less likely you are to get an organ transplant.

Finally, remember those aneurysms? Similarly, the blood vessels in your kidneys can pop, and when they do, it's deadly. Since your entire blood supply passes through your kidneys, if the blood vessels in your kidneys pop, you could die from massive internal bleeding.

Brain Damage

As we already discussed, high blood pressure puts you at an increased risk of stroke, the effects of which (assuming you survive) can include paralysis and memory loss.

You are also at a greater risk for dementia. This risk can come as a result of not having enough oxygen being delivered to the brain, which can also result in impairment to your brain that keeps you from being able to process information. The earlier in life that you begin to experience high blood pressure, the greater the damage will become as you age.[3]

Problems in the Bedroom

Believe it or not, hypertension is actually one of the most common causes of erectile dysfunction in men. Remember, high blood pressure affects all the blood vessels in the body, which includes the possibility of decreased flow to the penis. It also has the equivalent impact on women: blood flow to the vaginal area is critical for sexual arousal and satisfaction, and when one diminishes, so does the other. Treating high blood pressure often eliminates the need to take drugs, like Viagra® for sexual dysfunction. Your best bet for good sexual health is maintaining good heart health.

But another thing that happens in the bedroom gets affected, too. Studies note that high blood pressure and sleep apnea go hand in hand.

Sleep apnea keeps you from getting enough sleep and actually puts you at risk for heart disease and other problems.

Eye Opening Issues

Your eyes are very sensitive to changes in your blood pressure. The blood vessels of the eyes are very small and fragile, which makes them particularly vulnerable to the kind of damage we've been talking about. When the retina is not properly supplied with blood, it can lead to blurred (or even a complete loss of) vision if left unchecked.

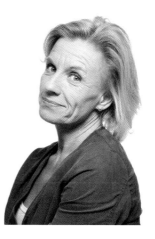

If you also have the secondary condition of diabetes, you're particularly at risk for this type of problem. Diabetes and high blood pressure greatly increase your risk of eye disease and loss of sight.

The Blood Pressure Solution

Additionally, you could face blockage in the blood vessels leading to your optic nerve. This, too, can lead to permanent blurred vision, and even blindness. It is critical that you pay attention to your blood pressure to maintain good vision.

Finally, ongoing high blood pressure can cause a buildup of fluid in your eye. The excess pressure this creates can cause damage and scarring inside the eye, which can lead to permanent vision deterioration.

Bad to the Bone

You might be surprised to know that you can even suffer from bone loss as a result of hypertension. People with high blood pressure lose more calcium, and as calcium leaves the bones and enters the bloodstream, bones can be left weak and brittle. The loss of calcium increases your risk for both osteoporosis and broken bones. In fact, most hip fractures in seniors are actually a result of bone disease.

While men can suffer from osteoporosis, women are generally more at risk after menopause. It is important to keep track of your blood pressure, and take corrective action whenever necessary.

CHAPTER 3

Causes Of High Blood Pressure

Your blood pressure naturally fluctuates to some degree, even when just walking into the doctor's office, especially if you're nervous. It might naturally begin to increase as you age, because your blood vessels become more rigid and inflexible. Generally, it doesn't change too much unless you're suffering from a condition that is highly correlated to having high blood pressure.

Here are some common risk factors:

- Overweight individuals have more instances of hypertension.

- Changing hormones can affect your blood pressure levels.

- Genetics play a role in whether or not you have hypertension.

- Stress and anxiety can cause spikes in your blood pressure.

- Diabetics experience more instances of high blood pressure.

- Too much salt (sodium) is a contributing factor to high blood pressure readings.

- The shape of your blood vessels will help or hurt your blood pressure.

- If your kidneys are in bad shape, this can cause high blood pressure.

- Smokers receive a diagnosis of hypertension more often than non- smokers. Overloading on alcohol can also cause high blood pressure readings.

- A deficiency in potassium and/or vitamin D can contribute to hypertension.

- African Americans tend to have a higher risk of hypertension.[1]

The medical community classifies high blood pressure into two broad categories: Primary and Secondary Hypertension.

Primary hypertension is diagnosed when doctors are unable to determine a specific medical condition that could be to blame for your high blood pressure. This is the case in about nine out of ten diagnoses of hypertension.

Secondary hypertension occurs when a specific medical condition, like kidney disease, causes the high blood pressure.

However, this doesn't mean that you can't do anything about it. In fact, it's just the opposite. It points to something I call "Lifestyle Induced High Blood Pressure," meaning that it was lifestyle choices that brought about the problem.

Believe it or not, this is great news!

It means that you are in complete control of it. If hypertension came as a result of specific choices you've made, all you have to do is appropriately modify your lifestyle, and you'll achieve better results. You can get rid of high blood pressure and avoid all the negative health issues that come with it.

Can Skinny People Have High Blood Pressure?

Let's clear a few things up right off the bat. First of all, we tend to assume that people with high blood pressure are overweight people. I mean, we look at them and just KNOW that all that weight is putting pressure on their arteries (correct or not). But don't be fooled by that — thin people can have issues as well.

As you will see, having higher blood sugar is a key foundational issue with blood pressure, and 20% of diabetics are thin. You don't have to be fat to have a blood sugar issue and you also don't have to be overweight to have a blood pressure issue. As you've seen (or will see) in this book, there are multiple issues involved with blood pressure, and while weight can affect blood pressure, you shouldn't assume that lack of weight automatically gives you health.

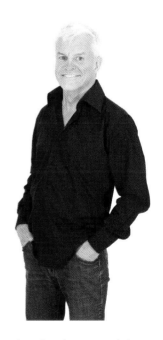

The Blood Pressure Solution

I remember a patient coming in, who lamented that her skinny friend was so healthy. And I said, "How do you know? Have you seen her blood tests?" Surprised, the patient looked at me, and I explained that you could have all sorts of health issues that don't show up on the outside. While losing weight can be helpful for blood pressure issues, that may not be enough. And in the same line of thinking, a thin person shouldn't try to lose weight if they have a blood pressure issue, as weight is probably not what's causing the problem.

Secondary Causes of High Blood Pressure

There are also other reasons that someone might have hypertension besides the more common ones we're discussing here. For example, kidney disease is one of the main reasons of secondary hypertension. You can also get hypertension from several different hormonal issues, like Cushing's disease, hyper- and hypothyroidism, and hyperparathyroidism (among others). Sleep apnea can absolutely be a cause, as can interactions (or side effects) of some medications.

But of all these issues, one thing is abundantly clear—it's not the salt.

The Sodium Dilemma

You may think you know something about how sodium affects your blood pressure, but believe me, it's actually way more complicated than you'd imagine.

Most people think of sodium as common table salt. I remember growing up and watching people gather around the kitchen table and apply very generous helpings of salt to almost everything on their plate.

If we had stuck to that, none of us would have gotten into trouble. The problem is, table salt actually has very little impact on our sodium intake—a 1991 study saw that 77% of sodium intake came from processed foods, while only 5% came from what was added during cooking, and 6% from what was added at the table.[2]

> {... 77% of sodium intake came from processed foods ...while only 6% was added at the table.}

When I say processed foods, I'm not just talking about the salty chips you're thinking of, but everything from spaghetti sauce, to bread, to processed meats, to soda. Since many people these days don't cook much at home and rely either on eating out or eating things that come out of bags, boxes, and cans, we have become a culture that consumes sodium in massive quantities.

Now it turns out that water is highly attracted to sodium. So wherever there is sodium in your body, water is sure to follow. This is why when you eat too many salty foods you start to feel bloated—sodium makes your body retain water. And since blood is over 50% water, when your sodium intake goes up, your blood volume goes up. The impact on your blood pressure will be almost immediate.

But you can't eliminate sodium from your diet altogether, because we very much need it to survive. Our bodies use sodium for cellular communication, which allows for proper muscle contraction and regulation of bodily fluids. So the key is to get your sodium intake under control and into healthy ranges.

Those healthy ranges are actually higher than you think—you may have heard for decades about low sodium being the key to hypertension, but the case for eating low sodium is actually on pretty shaky ground.

According to the newest research the ideal range for most people is between 2300 and 3000 mg per day, which is much higher than the 1500 mg recommended by the American Heart Association.

The newest studies are saying things like:

> "The Institute of Medicine recommends an intake of sodium of approximately 3800 mg of sodium chloride per day for adults 50 years of age or younger, approximately 3200 mg of sodium chloride per day for adults 51 to 70 years of age, and approximately 2900 mg of sodium chloride per day for those 71 years of age or older. The institute also

advises adults to consume at least approximately 4.7 g (or 4700 mg) of potassium per day, which is about twice the current U.S. average."[3] Probably not the recommendation you're getting from your doctor!

Or:

"...the committee found no evidence for benefit and some evidence suggesting risk of adverse health outcomes associated with sodium intake levels in ranges approximating 1,500 to 2,300 mg per day..."

Or this 2014 analysis of 25 studies that showed:

"Both low sodium intakes and high sodium intakes are associated with increased mortality."[4]

Another research paper indicated that people eating more than 7000 mg, or less than 3000 mg, had a higher rate of cardiovascular events like heart attacks.[5]

If you had low sodium intake and low blood pressure, that doesn't necessarily translate into less death or better survival rates, either. In fact, if your sodium or blood pressure levels get too low, your body's blood pressure actually increases!

More and more, we're seeing those low sodium guidelines linked with increased cardiovascular events,[6] increased

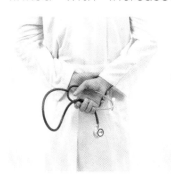

triglycerides and cholesterol,[7] insulin resistance (in as little as one week!),[6] and a higher risk of falls, broken hips, and decreased cognitive ability in the elderly.[7] If you're wondering why you haven't heard this from your doctor, this is because it

The Blood Pressure Solution

usually takes the research ten years to end up as medicinal recommendations according to several researchers I know personally. It's hard to let go of advice you've been giving for years.

The Truth About Salt

If you have high blood pressure, you have undoubtedly been told to limit your salt. You don't add salt to your food; you shy away from anything that is not labeled "low sodium", and probably regard salt as generally "bad." But it's not that simple to say salt is "good" or "bad."

One thing to keep in mind is that salt is so vital for human health that "sal-" is the basis of the word "salary" because people used to be paid in salt. Sodium and chloride are both vital minerals, used for nerve transmission/impulse conduction, fluid balance, and muscle contraction. Not having enough sodium will cause hyponatremia, a life-threatening condition that happens when someone sweats out too much sodium, or drinks too much water, and upsets the fluid balance.

Salt is a prime determinant for taste in food (along with fat) and *80% of the salt we consume is in processed foods,* making it difficult to avoid. The message promoted by both the National Heart, Lung, and Blood Institute (NHLBI) and the National High Blood Pressure Education Program (NHBPEP), a coalition of 36 medical organizations and six federal agencies, is that everyone, not just people will hypertension, would benefit from a daily intake of 2300 mg or sodium (6 grams of salt, or about 1 teaspoon) per day, which is over 1,000 mg less than our current average.

The problem lies in the fact that the research does not conclusively show that a reduction helps with blood pressure, and actually shows that low levels could lead to health problems. "You can say without any shadow of a doubt," says Drummond Rennie, an editor for the *Journal of the American Medical Association* and a physiologist at the University of California, "that the NHLBI has made a commitment to salt education that goes way beyond the scientific facts."[8]

You've probably noticed some of this—every once in a while, another article pops up in the newspaper, pointing out that low salt increases risk of mortality,[9, 10] increases heart disease or doesn't have any impact on lowering blood pressure,[11, 12] or even causes health issues like insulin resistance![5] And it's frustrating! Your doctor says one thing, but the research says another.

And these aren't insignificant research studies done on mice. A 2013 report which was compiled by a committee commissioned by the Institute of Medicine at the behest of the Centers for Disease Control and Prevention, said flat-out that there was no reason for ANYONE to aim for sodium levels under 2,300 mg per day, saying that not only was there no evidence indicating that it was helpful, but there were actually indications of possible harms—including increased rates of heart attacks and an increased risk of death.[12] And this was looking at only the newer research since 2005. The older research says this, as well.

Quite a few of the newer studies were focused on intakes of sodium at typically higher ranges (like 7,000 mg per day, with a lower end of 3,000 mg), and seeing that less than that could cause harm. The average person's intake is about

3,000 mg per day. This is in stark contrast to the American Heart Association, who doesn't just think 1,500 mg per day is enough, but thinks that EVERYONE should be maintaining such a low level, even though there's no evidence that this increases health, and can actually harm your health.

Now, it may be that perhaps the intake of someone who is genetically salt sensitive needs to be at a bit lower level, but nowhere as low as under the 2,300 mg per day. Instead, make adjustments in other areas of your life, which we'll talk about here; some with food, some with lifestyle, and see how much your blood pressure changes!

The Genetics of Salt Sensitivity

Yes, it's true; there is such a thing as having a genetic tendency to salt sensitivity, which can translate into hypertension. But here's the thing—most of the time, people DON'T react to salt. Let me explain.

There are many ways to determine if a person is salt-sensitive or salt-resistant, all of them involving an intake of sodium and measuring if someone's blood pressure rises in the aftermath.

One of the methods involves eating a low-sodium diet (about 230 mg sodium or 600 mg of table salt per day) for four days, followed by four days of a high-sodium diet (about 4.6 g sodium or 12 g of table salt per day). If blood pressure increases by at least 5% at the end of the high-sodium period, the person is said to be salt-sensitive. Otherwise, he or she is salt-resistant or salt-insensitive.[13] There are other versions of this test as well, but you get the picture.

There is no single gene that causes salt-sensitivity, as much as we'd like an easy answer. I once had a researcher say it takes the involvement of about a thousand genes to cause cancer. And while I don't know if that's fully accurate, it's definitely true that no single gene has been isolated for salt sensitivity. Yes, we've mapped the human genome, but we are nowhere close to figuring out which ones are involved and how they work together. Just to give you a sense of it, this 2011 paper on PubMed mentions over 25 different genes, some interacting with each other, or behaving differently in different populations, or the research showed something in mice but not in humans; and there are also variations of these genes that have different actions.[14]

Salt sensitivity has been found to be more prevalent in young, old, normotensive, and hypertensive African Americans compared to Caucasians, but even that is unclear in regards to genetics. They've done studies on this and found that salt sensitivity is so prevalent that it is considered to be a "hallmark" of hypertension for African Americans, as salt sensitivity is found in 73% of all African American hypertensive patients.[15]

Here's the issue, though—if it were just due to genetics, then we would see this in the African population, as well. But we don't. An international study of seven West African populations saw a prevalence of 33% in the U.S. but as low as 18% in West Africa.[16] That 18% rate of hypertension is lower even than for Caucasians in the U.S.! As one researcher says, "research indicates that one genetic hypothesis is insufficient to explain the relationship of salt sensitivity and blood pressure in African Americans. It is argued that race is a social (rather than biologic) concept, and that factors

The Blood Pressure Solution

other than biologic or genetic ones are responsible for the racial differences noted."[17]

Researchers have found that salt-sensitive people respond 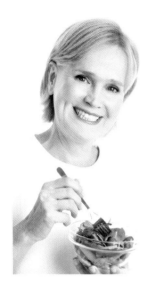 differently, not just to sodium, but also to other dietary factors. For example, salt-sensitive people excrete more calcium than others and adding calcium into a diet that has normal sodium intake can drop blood pressure.[18] Potassium is another one—low levels cause sodium retention and increased blood pressure, especially among African American men. The best source of potassium is found in fruits and vegetables, so eat up![19]

Like I mentioned before, salt reduction isn't helpful for the majority of people who aren't salt-sensitive, and can definitely cause harm, which is why over-reaching recommendations for everyone to reduce their sodium intake are problematic.

Salt Added to Food

Because we've heard again and again that limiting salt intake will help us with our blood pressure, some of us are more likely to use "no-salt" versions on our scrambled eggs in the morning, and to avoid adding salt when we're cooking. The problem is that this is typically not where the salt intake problem lies.

Our intake of processed foods has only increased since this study was done. So if you really wanted to moderate your salt intake, the key thing to do would be to eliminate eating things that come in bags, boxes, and cans, and reduce your eating out.

The bottom line is, don't worry about the saltshaker at the stove or at the table, and instead focus on sodium on the nutrition label and other dietary changes.

One of those changes, by the way, could be to use sea salt instead of regular table salt. We'll talk more about this in the section on Smart Supplementation in Chapter 5, but sea salt has a much better balance of minerals, like potassium, magnesium, and trace minerals, which are critical for managing blood pressure. Most individuals with hypertension have a deficiency or imbalance of these minerals, so adding them back in to your diet can really help.

Blood Sugar and Blood Pressure

We're so used to hearing how salt is the demon that causes blood pressure issues, that it doesn't really occur for us to consider that something else might actually be even MORE damaging. But in 2014, researchers published a paper titled, "The Wrong White Crystals: Not Salt But Sugar as Etiological in Hypertension and Cardiometabolic Disease."[20] They noted that while historically the focus of public health initiatives is always on salt, reducing salt intake typically only changes blood pressure by not much more than 4.8 mm Hg systolic and 2.5 mm Hg diastolic, and furthermore, they concluded that ingesting amounts less than 3,000 mg per day or more than 6,000 mg per day is associated with an increased risk of death and cardiovascular events.[21, 22, 23]

Additionally, they confirmed that processed foods are the primary source of dietary sodium, and that these harmful, manufactured foods are also among the leading sources of highly refined carbohydrates and sugar. Studies proved that sugar clearly causes hypertension. Exactly how much is insulin resistance related to hypertension? 80% of individuals with insulin resistance have hypertension, while only 25% of the population does.[24] Compared to non-diabetics, more diabetics have hypertension, and this is independent of being overweight.[25] In a study of over 2,700 people in both the USA and the UK, drinking sugar-sweetened beverages saw increased blood pressure having nothing to do with weight. The evidence goes on and on.[26]

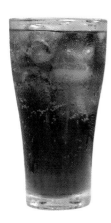

How does sugar cause high blood pressure? There are actually several mechanisms. Feeding sugar to rats increases their heart rate, sodium retention, vascular resistance, and renin secretion, all of which increase blood pressure. It also stimulates the sympathetic nervous system (the "flight or fight" reaction), which increases blood pressure. And they've seen this exact result in animal studies: eating sugar causes increased blood pressure.[27, 28, 29]

On a direct level, glucose in your bloodstream causes it to retain water. So if you eat a candy bar, your blood sugar goes up, and in turn, your blood pressure automatically increases. However, that increase will only be temporary, and when your blood sugar goes back down so will your blood pressure.

On the surface that doesn't sound so bad, though it is problematic for reasons we'll get to in a minute. But when we consider the long-term effects sugar has, it gets much, much worse.

All of your cells use glucose for energy. But glucose can't enter the cells on its own, it needs a chaperone to unlock your cell membrane and shepherd it in. That chaperone is insulin. When your tongue tastes something sweet, your brain says, "Ooh, sugar!" and sends a message to your pancreas to release insulin into your bloodstream.

"I thought salt was the worst thing for blood pressure!" I hear those words all the time. And while we've seen that there's *some* truth to that, for most people *SUGAR* is a much more important factor.

The problem is that when you eat sugar all the time, your body continuously thinks, "Ooh, this is the time of year when sugar is available!" Keep in mind that 100,000 years ago we only got sugar at certain times of year when fruits, and the few carb-heavy vegetables, were plentiful. Your body anticipates that you're *about* to eat sugar even before you actually eat it, and in response, it dumps insulin into the bloodstream. This pulls out all the sugar that's currently in there, which means now your blood sugar is lower than necessary to perform your basic body functions. This makes you crave more sugar and prevents you from burning fat (since, obviously, you need to store fat at this time of year while food is plentiful in anticipation of the winter when food is scarce).

The cravings lead people to eat something carb-heavy in order to use up that insulin and restore your blood sugar to its "baseline minimum." But eating that carb-heavy food then spikes your blood sugar. Since, after twenty or thirty or sixty years of doing this these cravings are constant, our bodies are in a perpetual blood sugar roller-coaster, spending half its time in a crash and half its time in a spike, increasing your blood pressure every time your sugar level spikes. Over time, this doesn't do great things to the walls of your arteries.

But also, after years of this, the cells start to become desensitized to the presence of insulin. This means that the glucose can't get into all those cells, and instead it continues to float around the bloodstream. Your body responds by removing the glucose from the bloodstream and turning it into fat. It's the process of converting sugar into fat that produces triglycerides.

If this process continues unchecked, the eventual result is a chronic disease of some sort: heart disease, cancer, cerebrovascular disease, Alzheimer's, and diabetes—which happen to be five of the seven leading causes of death in the United States,[30] and all are driven in large part by this exact problem. And often, these diseases coincide.

To give just one example, according to the American Diabetics Association, 71% of diabetics are also hypertensive.[31] Keep in mind, it's not that one leads to the other, but rather it's the *same thing* that causes both.

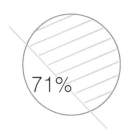

71% of All Diabetics Also Have High Blood Pressure

And believe it or not, this actually gets worse if you're adding fructose into the mix – not to mention high fructose corn syrup.

So far we've talked just about glucose. All carbohydrates break down into glucose, so it doesn't matter if it's a potato, or rice, or whole wheat bread, or something else that's theoretically nutritious. The carbs are going to have this impact on your body.

But fructose has to be processed in the liver before the cells can use it. And the process of converting fructose into glucose produces triglycerides at a much higher rate that consuming straight glucose does.[32]

You know what table sugar is? Sucrose—which is a glucose molecule and a fructose molecule stuck together (i.e., 50% fructose and 50% glucose). You know what high fructose corn syrup is? It's a mixture that's about 55/45. How about honey? It's mostly just fructose, glucose, sucrose, and water. And how does agave nectar compare? It comes in at between 60 and 95% fructose, depending on the brand. And maple syrup? I think you get the point.

Simply put, sugar puts glucose into the bloodstream, which spikes blood pressure in the short-term, and causes insulin resistance, which spikes blood pressure in the long-term. And since sodium is so valuable for the body and sugar is so bad for it, I would focus all my efforts on getting my sugar intake under control before I would start to worry about salt.

So if you wanted to make an impact on your blood pressure, this is the very first place to start. But where do *you* start?

I've actually written a separate book about this, but the first step is to get a sense of how many carbohydrates you eat, as those all convert into glucose (which then triggers insulin). Now, many carbohydrates are really good for you, like vegetables, and whole grains. But depending on how long you've been eating the "bad ones" (like white bread, cereal, and "coffee dessert" drinks from your local barista), you may or may not be able to tolerate all of these, it just depends.

What I typically do in my clinical practice is tell people to use a website like www.myfitnesspal.com, or www.loseit.com, or any of the other online sources or apps out there, and total up the carbohydrate intake of the foods and drinks they consume, but ONLY those from this list:

- Bread
- Crackers/Chips
- Cereal/Granola/Bran
- Breakfast Bars/Granola Bars/Energy Bars
- Oatmeal
- Rice
- Candy
- Baked Goods
- Pastries
- Cookies/Cakes
- Fruit Juices
- Energy Drinks
- Milk
- Soda
- Alcoholic Beverages
- Fruit
- Beans
- Potatoes/Sweet Potatoes
- Corn (including popcorn)

This does *not* include green vegetables, or foods like beets or carrots, since, as I often say, "No one gets diabetes or hypertension from carrots!" You'll have to check for two things—the grams of carbohydrates of the food and the serving size. Make sure to actually measure your serving size, as we will often take more than that without realizing it. You don't need to write down anything but the carbohydrate number— not added sugars (it's already contained in the carbohydrate number), nor fats or proteins. Just carbohydrates. Write these down for about 4-5 days, and total them up. What did you get?

{"No one gets diabetes or hypertension from eating carrots!"}

If you're calculating carbs from items on the above list, we're shooting for a total of about 60g per day. Remember, this doesn't include green vegetables, or vegetables like beets or carrots. Just the things from the list. How did you do?

The average person usually has about 300-800g of carbohydrates per day. Importantly, just imagine every time you're eating a carbohydrate, (especially one that is filled with white flour and sugar), that when you eat it, it causes all of the things we mentioned above—all of them resulting in high blood pressure. That's why we say this is the first place to start.

Remember those researchers we mentioned before? The ones who wrote that research paper, saying that sugar, not salt, was the instigator of high blood pressure? This is what they wrote in their conclusion:

"...While there is no argument that recommendations to reduce consumption of processed foods are highly appropriate and advisable, the arguments in this review are that the benefits of such recommendations might have less to do with sodium—minimally related to blood pressure and perhaps even inversely related to cardiovascular risk—and more to do with highly-refined carbohydrates. It is time for guideline committees to shift focus away from salt and focus greater attention to the likely more-consequential food additive: sugar."

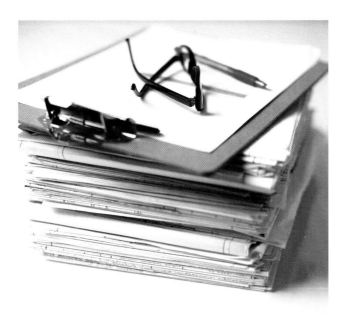

CHAPTER 4

The Healthcare Industry's Answer to High Blood Pressure

Most people are diagnosed with hypertension during a routine office visit with their family doctor. If this happened to you, you were probably told to stop eating salt, exercise more, and you might have been prescribed a few specific medications.

To be clear, some people need to be on prescription drugs to control their high blood pressure. However, many people do not and can control their blood pressure without the need for medications, (most of which being not only expensive but often come with unpleasant side effects).

Before we even talk about those, I should stress that it's never a bad idea to monitor your blood pressure readings for a period of a week or so to determine the average of your blood pressure readings.[1]

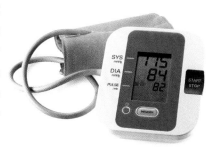

The Blood Pressure Solution

A single high reading isn't usually a cause for alarm (unless it is dangerously high and requires immediate medical attention), so if this is the first time you've ever been told you have high blood pressure, go buy a blood pressure cuff from your nearest pharmacy, and take a reading once or twice a day for at least a few days.

If you are you using an app on your smart phone that helps you track health information, know that these can be very helpful sometimes, as they help track diet, exercise, water intake, etc., and some even share the information with your doctor. But be careful—some of the apps claim to be able to accurately measure your blood pressure by using your finger pressed against the phone camera. I don't know about you, but I don't feel that we're at that point yet of feeling confident in the accuracy of results from testing your blood pressure using a phone camera. I wouldn't trust your health to such an unreliable device.

A 2015 research study looked at the top 107 apps designed for blood pressure management and found that less than 3% of them were developed by healthcare agencies (such as a university or professional organization), and none of them used a BP cuff or have any documentation showing it's effectiveness against a gold standard.[2]

Until these are better developed, do yourself a favor, and stick to the accurate monitors that you know will give you the correct picture of your blood pressure.

As far as doctor recommended treatments are concerned, a treatment plan will often include an ACE inhibitor and a beta-blocker, along with other medications, that are adjusted to the individual patient's needs.[3]

The Blood Pressure Solution

Here is a list of the most common high blood pressure medications, traditionally prescribed by the medical community:

ACE Inhibitors

How They Work: This type of drug blocks the creation of a specific chemical in your body that causes your blood vessels to constrict. Without this chemical, your blood vessels relax and allow blood to flow more easily than before.

Side effects include: Hypotension, an irritating dry cough, headache, dizziness, fatigue, nausea, and renal impairment.

Alpha Blockers

How They Work: Alpha-blockers also help with relaxing the blood vessels so that blood can flow more easily.

Side effects include: Dizziness (from rapid decreases in blood pressure), headache, pounding heartbeat, nausea, weakness, and weight gain.

Beta Blockers

How They Work: These drugs block naturally occurring epinephrine, also known as adrenaline. This has the effect of keeping your heart rate slower and pumping with less force, thereby pushing less blood through your system and lowering blood pressure.

Side effects include: Fatigue, cold hands, headache, upset stomach, constipation, diarrhea, and dizziness.

Diuretics

How They Work: Diuretics flush water out of your body. Since blood is made up of about 50% water, this process reduces the volume of blood. The water also takes much of the salt with it, which helps to reduce blood pressure.

Side effects: Weakness, dizziness, blurred vision, headache, fever, sore throat, ringing in ears, skin rash, nausea, and even heart palpitations. Unfortunately a diuretic cannot distinguish between the different minerals in your bodily fluid, so it also flushes out many of the beneficial ones like potassium, leading to muscle cramps. Other side effects include weakness, dizziness, blurred vision, headache, fever, sore throat, ringing in ears, skin rash, nausea, and even heart palpitations.

Vasodilators

How They Work: Vasodilators open your blood vessels up to create more interior room for proper blood flow. This lowers the pressure inside the blood vessel due to the extra room created by the expansion.

Side effects: Rapid heartbeat, headaches, dizziness, nausea, vomiting, bloating, sore throat, joint pain, swollen feet or legs, flushing (similar to the sensations of blushing, but typically more pronounced), swollen lymph nodes, fever, skin blisters, or itching.

4 Worst Blood Pressure Drugs

Lisinopril

Lisinopril's side effects include nausea, vomiting, kidney failure, and even heart attacks. The last one is especially alarming, because it is one of the very things the drug is supposed to *prevent.* As an ACE inhibitor, lisinopril is supposed to block a natural enzyme that tightens blood vessels, forcing the blood vessels to open wider, thus lowering blood pressure and your risk for heart attacks.

Due to the overwhelming prevalence of these reactions, lisinopril has received 406,180 complaints to the FDA in less than 10 years. That's over 40,000 complaints per year and over 110 complaints *per day.*

Lisinopril can also cause a rapid loss of blood pressure that makes you swoon with dizziness or even pass out. You might be shocked to hear that ACE inhibitors are derived from the venom of the Brazilian Pit Viper. I know you might be wondering, "What on earth does snake venom have to do with treating high blood pressure?" Well, it's understandable when you learn that this snake's venom causes a rapid loss of blood pressure in the snake's prey, knocking them out so that they can be easily consumed. The same thing can happen to lisinopril users, especially when they stand up after sitting for a while. This can cause a serious fall, leading to broken hips and fractured skulls.

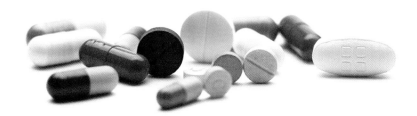

It is a good thing that many doctors are refusing to prescribe this drug to their older patients, but others are worried about letting their patients walk around with high blood pressure, increasing their risk of a stroke. This makes for a difficult trade-off. Many doctors are faced with choosing between putting their patients at risk for a stroke or putting them at risk for a serious fall that can end their walking days. This is especially difficult because doctors know that a fall can be just as fatal as a stroke.

But even if you don't get dizzy from lisinopril, you've got a good chance of developing a persistent cough that won't go away. You see, drugs don't just disappear after you've stopped taking them. Your body still has to break them down over a certain period of time (that can vary person to person). This becomes a problem when a person's kidneys can't filter a byproduct of lisinopril, called "kinins." When this happens, kinins can become trapped in the lungs, so that the only way to expel them is to cough them up.

Some studies show that up to one-third of lisinopril users suffer from this cough,[4] and for some, the cough doesn't go away when the drug is stopped. Keep in mind, we're not talking about just a "little cough", either. It has been reported that people have coughed so hard that they have vomited, passed out, or busted ribs.

Metoprolol Succinate

Over forty million prescriptions for metoprolol succinate are filled every year, and 90% of these are generic. Most of these generic drugs are manufactured outside the U.S., where oversight is lax, and tiny changes creep into the manufacturing process, which can interfere with how the drug is supposed to work.

The FDA is finally cracking down on this drug after *thousands* of patients *and* doctors have flooded the federal agency with angry calls and letters. The alarming thing is that, these complaints are for the *generic* version of the drug, which is supposed to be identical to the brand name only more affordable, right? It turns out, that's not the case.

Metoprolol succinate just isn't safe. Whether generic or name brand, it can still cause nausea, dizziness, difficulty in breathing, and it can reduce your strength and make you feel very weak.

As a "beta-blocker," metoprolol succinate blocks adrenaline from working in your body (remember, it's the hormone that governs the body's "fight or flight" responses). When you have less adrenaline, the force and speed of your heart beat is reduced, which can lower blood pressure.

But sometimes we need adrenaline, like when we're facing a critical decision at work, or even something as seemingly simple as needing to change lanes quickly while driving. And when we don't get that surge, we feel sluggish, unsteady, and just plain fragile.

I know this not only from the research, by from personal experience, as well. I was prescribed a beta-blocker for a heart condition, and it robbed me of energy, which made it even more difficult to get back to cycling.

Amlodipine

Amlodipine is notorious for causing side effects like headache, hair loss, and embarrassing diarrhea. It also reduces aldosterone (the water retention hormone) production, which can cause frequent urination, sweating, a slightly higher body temperature, and feeling dehydrated. What's even scarier is that, it can cause emotional disturbances like depression, panic attacks, and suicidal thoughts. This drug is also responsible for causing painful swelling in the ankles and wrists that are bad enough to leave you bed-ridden.

As a "calcium channel blocker," amlodipine lowers blood pressure by interfering with the electrical signals in your muscles. It acts like an insulator, which slows nerve signals, weakens contractions in the heart and arteries. By slowing down these contractions, your blood vessels can't tighten as much, which in turn, lowers your blood pressure.

However, by tampering with the integrity of your blood vessels, amlodipine permits fluid from blood to rush into otherwise healthy tissue, especially the tissue surrounding your ankles and wrists. This can result is painful swelling that can make it very difficult to walk.

The Blood Pressure Solution

Chlorothiazide

Chlorothiazide increases your risk of painful muscle cramping, paralysis, seizure, slipping into a coma, and in some cases, it can interfere your heart rhythm so badly that your heart can actually just stop beating.

As a "diuretic" or "water pill," chlorothiazide works by flushing water out of your system, and with less water in your body, there is less pressure in your blood vessels.

However, while diuretics flush water out of your body, they can also flush out vital nutrients like electrolytes, which your body needs to keep your heart rhythm normal and your muscles working.

As you have probably realized, these medications try to manipulate all seven of the exact same variables identified in the first part of this book. They can have some serious side effects, and though they work as a short-term solution, they don't address the root cause of your high blood pressure at all, which means that you will probably have to take those drugs, and live with those side effects, for the rest of your life.

Wouldn't it be better for us if there were some healthier way to lower our blood pressure naturally?

Yes!

Why deal with those side effects when you can just as easily, and far less expensively, lower your blood pressure with some simple dietary and lifestyle changes?

That is exactly what I am about to teach you how to do!

Warning: Don't Stop Your Prescriptions Without Talking To Your Doctor

Again, I want to be very clear here, I am not recommending you stop taking any blood pressure medication that you are currently taking. Instead, I suggest you talk to your doctor about your desire to lower your blood pressure naturally. Ask him to look over your plan and help you transition into coming off of your blood pressure drugs in a way that does not harm your health.

However, if you aren't on any of these drugs yet, then I want to encourage you to keep reading. With the information I am about to share, you will finally have the knowledge necessary to control your high blood pressure using natural cures.

CHAPTER 5

The Blood Pressure Solution: Lower Your Blood Pressure Naturally!

The Blood Pressure Solution Program is based on the idea that blood pressure is something that can be controlled naturally through smart changes to diet and lifestyle.

To that end, we will be tackling your hypertension on many fronts, all of which are proven to positively improve a person's blood pressure.

As you begin to implement these strategies you will quickly realize how interrelated the causes and cures to high blood pressure really are.

Consider the Seven Blood Pressure Levers:

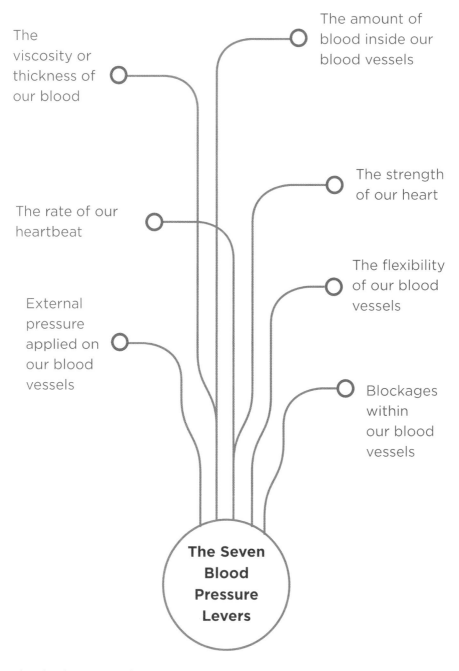

The viscosity or thickness of our blood

The amount of blood inside our blood vessels

The strength of our heart

The rate of our heartbeat

The flexibility of our blood vessels

External pressure applied on our blood vessels

Blockages within our blood vessels

The Seven Blood Pressure Levers

The Blood Pressure Solution

All the adjustments we're about to give you work together synergistically. One change impacts multiple levers. So the more of them you implement, the greater the effect.

For example: as you cut certain foods out and add others in, you may lose weight. The loss of weight takes pressure off the outside walls of your blood vessels and reduces blood pressure independently of the effect those dietary changes would have had all on their own. The reduction of processed foods also reduces sodium intake, which releases extra water and with it the volume of blood. Eating less sugar and flour also reduces the amount of insulin your body needs, which also reduces that extra water, since insulin causes fluid retention. Essentially, as you begin to eat smarter and exercise more, you will also start to repair the damaged blood vessels, improving their flexibility.

This is just the tip of the iceberg. The key point I want to make here is that this is a system where the whole is much, much more than just the sum of its parts. Every change you make impacts everything else. And when you make these changes together, they work with each other, increasing and compounding the benefits.

Now remember, these are the same seven levers that the medical community tries to manipulate as well, but they're using a different approach, by prescribing drugs that have many unwanted side effects. Modifying these levers naturally will get similar (if not the same) results, but with few or no side effects.

There are six categories we'll be looking at:

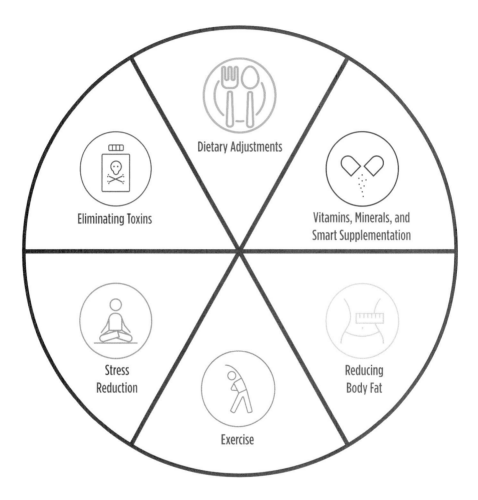

Here we go.

Category 1: Dietary Adjustments

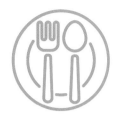

When I was diagnosed with that heart condition, the first thing my doctor did was give me a prescription for a beta-blocker. If you remember, beta-blockers slow your heart rate down, which makes you tired, among other symptoms. I was desperate to come off of them, but I didn't know what else to do.

One of the first things that other doctor—the one who was actually interested in nutrition—told me to do was to cut out the "bad food", and eat healthy foods. Simply put, he told me to eat "real food", and eliminate foods that were heavily processed and full of chemicals, sodium, and sugar, which are harmful for your metabolism and your immune system.

In retrospect, it sounds kind of obvious. Eat things that our ancestors could have eaten. Don't eat things that were invented in a laboratory. However, in our culture, we're not really taught to do that.

So let's start by looking at the macronutrients and what we *should* be eating, and then we'll come back to look at the ones to cut out.

A Macronutrient Primer

When you consume food you are essentially putting raw nutrients into your body. Your body will then take these raw nutrients and use some of them for energy, some of them for building muscle and other tissues, and some of them to help create the hormones and other biochemistry needed to properly operate your body.

All food falls into one or more of the three main macronutrient types: carbohydrates, fats, and protein.

Carbohydrates

Typically used for energy, carbohydrates are found in fruits, vegetables, nuts, and many processed foods. All carbohydrates break down into glucose in your bloodstream. Glucose is also known as "blood sugar", and your body uses this to provide energy to your cells. In order to get the glucose out of your bloodstream and into your cells, your body must release insulin into your bloodstream, as well. The unfortunate side effect of this is that the minute insulin spikes, fat storage begins.

Fats

Fats have gotten a bad rap in the mainstream press, but they're essential to your health. It has been proven that dietary fat does not make you produce body fat. Rather, it helps your brain function, provides a secondary energy source, protects your cells, and tells your body when you are full so that you don't overeat. You've no doubt heard about 'good' fats that come from avocados, coconut oil, extra virgin olive oil, and some nuts, but the same is true of the natural animal fats that come from beef, chicken, pork, fish, and dairy, all of which are perfectly fine.

With that in mind, here are some healthy fats that are perfectly fine to have in your diet:

The Blood Pressure Solution

- Fats in meat or dairy (including red meat and butter)

- Chicken skin

- Eggs

- Coconut oil

- Avocado

- Lard

- Seed oils (olive, peanut, sesame, etc.)

- Nuts and seeds

Now, I know what you're thinking already. Lard? How can that possibly be a healthy fat? Every time I mention this one, it never fails to shock people a bit. You've probably heard for years that the "lard clogs your pipes," but the truth is that lard is actually in the same kind of fat as olive oil—a monounsaturated fat. For this reason, it's really making a comeback as a good cooking oil. (For more information, I highly recommend the article, "Lard: The New Health Food," in *Food and Wine magazine*. It does a great job sorting out all the misinformation and misunderstandings about lard.)

Coconut oil is particularly helpful when you're changing your diet in the way we recommend. It's what's known as a "medium-chain fatty acid," meaning that your body is not going to store it as fat. Instead, your body uses it almost as if it was a carbohydrate—that means quick energy! You can use this oil whenever you're cooking your food, but we've also heard from our patients that they like to stir it into their coffee and tea for a quick pick-me-up, or even lick it off a spoon! You can buy this oil in two types: refined and unrefined. The refined kind doesn't taste like coconut like the unrefined does, but they both work the same. And don't worry, there's no weird chemistry in the refining process—it only means that they removed the coconut proteins. So pick whichever tastes better to you.

Now, here are some fats that should be AVOIDED:

- Partially hydrogenated vegetable fats (trans-fats)
- Unsaturated, processed vegetable oils that aren't expeller or cold pressed

Commercially prepared seed oils (corn, canola, vegetable, etc.) found in grocery stores are just not safe to eat. They use high temperatures and chemical solvents to economically extract the oils, and in the process the oils become damaged and rancid. The offensive smells are removed prior to bottling, but the free radicals are still present. These oils are one of the leading causes of heart disease.

Protein

Proteins are the building blocks of muscle and are essential to your diet. Without protein in your diet your muscles would waste away and you would eventually be unable to move.

The macronutrient ratio that I've found works very well in helping maintain high energy levels, lose weight, and still feel satisfied and not hungry during the day is: 65% Fat, 25% Protein, and 10% Carbs.

Daily Calorie Ratio

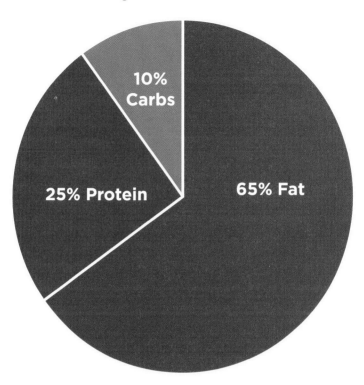

You may be stunned to read this graph. This is because we've been taught that fat is bad, and that to lose weight one must cut calories. Our current diabetes epidemic was caused in part by taking fat out of our diet and then overeating carbohydrates. You see, fat has several jobs in the body, including transporting minerals around and containing vitamins, so because of this, low fat diets can actually cause other issues as well. We're going to put balance back into your diet by reducing your carbohydrates and increasing your fat intake, which will have you feeling much better AND improve several health concerns.

So with that in mind, you can reach these targets from the following places:

Meat, Eggs, and Dairy

Animal products are most people's number one source for protein and fat. They're incredibly nutrient-dense and do a great job filling you up, especially when you **leave the fat on.** That really is key. So quit getting boneless skinless chicken breasts, and get the full chicken.

And also, switch out skim milk for whole. You'll feel fuller and get far more nutrients.

Examples:

- Beef (grass fed is best)
- Chicken (free range from local grower is best)
- Salmon (wild caught is best)
- Halibut (wild caught is best)
- Pork (if cured, make sure to find low sodium varieties)
- Bacon (low sodium cured)
- Eggs (I suggest organic or farm grown eggs)

Vegetables

Vegetables are nature's suppliers of many vital nutrients, both vitamins and minerals. It is always best to select vegetables from the list below, particularly those vegetables of the dark green, leafy variety, to get the most beneficial nutrients in your diet.

The Blood Pressure Solution

Examples:

- Spinach
- Chili Peppers
- Beets
- Broccoli
- Winter Squash
- Zucchini
- Kale

- Swiss Chard
- Brussels Sprouts
- Green Beans
- Asparagus
- Celery
- Carrots

Fruit

Fruits are a rich source of many antioxidants and other important vitamins and minerals, but it's easy to eat too much fruit, especially if you're trying to avoid sugar. As a guideline, I usually tell my patients, "Eat twice as many vegetables as fruits." The smaller fruits, like berries, have less sugar. I recommend the following fruits be on the top of your weekly shopping list:

Examples:

- Blueberries
- Strawberries
- Raspberries
- Avocados

- Melons
- Apples
- Whatever is in season!

Nuts and Seeds

Nuts and seeds are a great source of good fats, and will help you not only feel full, but provide great nutrient value, as well. Watch it on the sodium—if you like your nuts to be salted, either get the "lightly salted" kind, or buy both raw and salted nuts, and mix them together. It's easy to overeat nuts, so don't go crazy with them.

Examples:

- Pistachios
- Almonds
- Brazil Nuts
- Pumpkin Seeds
- Cashews

Spices

Herbs and spices are a healthy way to add flavor to your plate without adding sodium.

Examples (fresh or dried):

- Sage
- Thyme
- Oregano
- Cilantro
- Basil
- Mint
- Parsley
- Dill
- Garlic/Chives/Shallot/Onion

Oils

Healthy oils are another great source of fats. Whether used for cooking, marinades, or salad dressing, healthy oils are always beneficial. For these, always make sure you're getting naturally occurring oils like the ones listed below.

Examples:

- Coconut Oil
- Olive oil
- Butter
- Grape seed Oil
- Avocado oil

However, heavily processed oils—like corn oil, vegetable oil, and soy oil are really inflammatory. And anything with trans fats or hydrogenated fats—avoid at all costs as they are a disaster!

Herbal Teas

While you won't get any calories from herbal teas, you will get multiple benefits from the plant compounds and nutrients in them.

Examples:

- Hibiscus Tea
- Green Tea
- Oolong Tea
- Fruit Teas

The complete food list is included in the Bonus guide, "99 Foods That Naturally Lower Blood Pressure," which can be found by logging in to your Member's Area at: http://bloodpressuresolution.com/login/

Eating To Live

As I began to investigate nutrition and it's impact on health, I noticed a common theme. The vitamins, minerals, and other nutrient-based solutions were most readily accessible through either real foods, or in some cases, supplements. When I say real foods, I am talking about foods that have a single ingredient: bananas, raisins, grapes, spinach, etc.

Nowhere in the research are any processed foods recommended. This realization was a profound moment for me. The more I researched and understood the damaging impact that manufactured foods had on our bodies, the more I started to adopt a very simple way of eating. This style of eating predates the modern era and instead of providing your body with a bewildering array of chemical additives, instead it supplies your body with the foods it has thrived on for millennia. Just simple, natural, real food is all your body needs and wants.

Simply put, we have two options regarding the types of food we can put into our bodies: processed foods and natural foods.

Processed Foods

A manufactured food is something that that has been heavily processed in a factory and cannot be found in nature. This includes (but is not limited to):

- Bread
- Pasta

- Candies and desserts

- Instant mixes

- TV dinners

- Soft drinks, fruit juices, and energy drinks

- Foods that are skimmed, enhanced, enriched, or otherwise adulterated

- Processed vegetable oils, including canola, corn, and soybean

- Things that are fried and broiled at high temperatures

- Artificial sweeteners

- Hydrogenated or partially hydrogenated fats (trans fats)

- Energy bars, protein shakes, and other "health" foods

- Preservatives like benzoic acid

- Artificial additives, including dyes, preservatives, flavors (even "natural" flavors), MSG, etc.

If these "foods" ever had any nutrients in them, most or all of them are removed and replaced with chemical additives to provide taste and, often, to make them more addictive.[1] I know, this sounds like the stuff of conspiracy theorists, but manufactured foods bind to the chemical receptors in our brains in just the same way that drugs like cocaine or heroin do, making us crave them and want more of them—and then you wonder why you don't have the willpower to resist things you know are bad for you!

Typically, these foods are high—dangerously high—in sodium and/or sugar. This isn't just for the flavor. Both compounds also serve a number of other chemical functions—for example, improving texture, consistency, color, and even acting as a preservative. This is part of why you so often see sugar listed in the ingredients for things that you otherwise never would have expected like bread, or ketchup, or peanut butter.

These foods feed the bad bacteria in your gut—and since your gut bacteria actually account for roughly two-thirds of your immune system,[2] when those get out of balance, it can be a big problem. It leads to inflammation, toxins building up in your body, and your cells becoming undernourished, which means that, on a cellular level, your body isn't working the way it should. And then all of this gunk builds up inside your bloodstream, attracts water, and inflames everything in and around the walls of your blood vessels, which... you guessed it... increases the pressure on those arterial walls.

Note that hydrogenated oils play a particularly evil role in all of this. In addition to doing what you have read above, they also contain trans fats, which is like injecting the oil directly into your veins. And another note: even if the label says 0g trans fats, if it's got *hydrogenated oil* it's got trans fats in it—the companies just make sure to keep it under 0.5g so they can get away with saying that; but it adds up very quickly.

And one more note, on commercially prepared vegetable oils: corn, canola, vegetable, and soy are the common ones in this country. They use high temperatures and chemical solvents to economically extract the oils, and in the process the oils become damaged and rancid. The offensive smells are removed prior to bottling, but the free radicals are still present. These oils are one of the leading causes of heart disease. If you think about it, none of those foods are naturally very oily. So stick to oils that come from sources that are obviously fatty—peanut, tree nuts, avocado, coconut, and animal fats—and you'll be fine.

Natural (or Whole) Foods

These foods are made up of just one ingredient and typically are either an animal product, or something that grew from the ground. Things like fruits, vegetables, beef, chicken, fish, etc. Of course, when buying these foods, you have two options: organic and non-organic.

Organic vs. Non-Organic Foods

There's a lot of debate about whether or not buying organic produce is worth it. There are complaints about the cost, that the produce sometimes doesn't look as good, it's just a gimmick, etc. Here's the skinny on this topic:

Organic food is defined as being produced without the use of pesticides or man-made fertilizers, growth regulators or livestock feed additives. There are two main reasons that people might choose to eat organic. One is that a lot of people are uncomfortable ingesting chemicals into their bodies, especially since the chemical industry isn't regulated, as aggressively as many people would like. The second reason people eat organic is because the food they're eating has more nutritional value and therefore supports your health better.

For example, take that head of lettuce you were thinking of making into a salad later today. You might look up the nutritional value on the Internet, but how do you KNOW it contains what it says? The nutrition of a plant is dependent on the soil quality, and that soil quality has been known to be declining for years.[3] As I've said in lectures many times, we can't digest rocks. So we have the plants do it for us, and then we eat the plants! But if the soil is poor, then we might be eating that lettuce but not getting nearly as much nutrition as we thought.

Just like us, the plants need nourishment to have healthy immune systems and to be strong; and if the soil isn't good, they get weak and vulnerable. Which then leads to the use of pesticides and fertilizers, as the plant can't defend itself— and the soil, from over-farming, doesn't provide enough nutrition for the plant. And then we eat those plants, having no idea of where the plant came from or how it was grown, and assume a certain level of nutrition, which truthfully, I wouldn't assume, if I were you.

A 2014 study, a meta-analysis of 343 research articles on nutritional content and pesticide residue on organic and non-organic produce, found that "organic crops, on average, have higher concentrations of antioxidants, lower concentrations of Cadmium, and a lower incidence of pesticide residues than the non-organic comparators across regions and production seasons."[4] It saw that pesticide residue was four times higher in conventional crops, and saw statistically significant increases in the amounts of minerals and plant compounds that are known to have health effects.

The same is true for meat production. Organically raised meat is higher in Omega-3 fatty acids while conventionally, factory-farmed meat is higher in the more inflammatory Omega-6's, primarily because those animals are fed large amounts of corn, rather than the grass they would normally eat. Also, organic meat farmers do not use antibiotics to increase the weight of the animal, or hormones, or anything else unnatural, for that matter.

And here's a trick you can use immediately—this is a list of the Dirty Dozen (the 12 fruits and vegetables that you should buy organic if possible, as they have the highest pesticide residues) and the Clean Fifteen (the 15 foods that are clean enough to buy non-organic). Remember, this list is *only referring* to the pesticide residue and not to the nutritional content.

Dirty Dozen (buy organic):

Strawberries	Cherries
Apples	Spinach
Nectarines	Tomatoes
Peaches	Sweet Bell Peppers
Celery	Cherry Tomatoes
Grapes	Cucumbers

Each of these foods tested positive for a number of different pesticide residues and showed higher concentrations of pesticides than other produce.

The Blood Pressure Solution

Clean Fifteen:

Avocados	Onions	Eggplant
Sweet Corn	Asparagus	Honeydew Melon
Pineapples	Mangos	Grapefruit
Cabbage	Papayas	Cantaloupe
Sweet peas frozen	Kiwi	Cauliflower

For your health, and to get the most out of your food, the best option is to grow your own vegetables. If you can't do that, buy organic when you can, and buying local organic is even better!

A Word About the DASH Diet

You may have heard a lot about the DASH diet, which was created by the National Institutes of Health, and has won wide-ranging acclaim for its positive impact on lowering high blood pressure.

While it does have some very good suggestions—namely that it takes out processed foods, restricts sugar, and increases fresh vegetables and fruit—it still roughly follows the debunked Food Pyramid that was so boldly promoted by the U.S. government for years. The high carbohydrate recommendations, as well as the restriction of dietary fat, are a deal killer for me. I have witnessed firsthand the negative impact of consuming too many carbs from grain-based products, and I have also witnessed first hand the very positive health benefits that one can achieve from increasing the amount of fat in your diet. For that reason, I just can't wholeheartedly recommend the DASH diet.

Category 2: Vitamins, Minerals, and Smart Supplementation

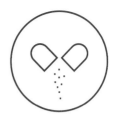

While I recommend getting as many of the blood pressure-lowering vitamins and minerals as you can from the foods you eat each day, sometimes that simply isn't possible. Modern farming techniques have actually reduced much of the nutrition out of our food, and certain things may be difficult or impossible for you to find. So in this section, I will outline exactly what vitamins, minerals, and herbs that I recommend to supplement your diet if you are serious about lowering your blood pressure. Each of these has been highly researched, and studies show that they work.

Vitamins, Minerals, and Smart Supplementation:

Vitamins

Vitamins can actually be broken down into two categories: water-soluble and fat-soluble. Water-soluble vitamins are easily absorbed into your body, and they are not stored for very long. Your body will flush out any excess amount of these vitamins. Therefore, it is important to replenish these vitamins, as often as possible.

Fat-soluble vitamins are absorbed into the small intestine and stored in the fatty tissues of the body. For this reason, there is never any reason to consume more than the daily-recommended dose of these vitamins.

Water-Soluble Vitamins

B6

It's hard to separate the effects of all the B vitamins from one another, so let's look at them in part and in whole. We will start with B6. True Vitamin B6 deficiency is rare outside of cases such as chronic alcoholism and frank malnutrition, but B6 *insufficiency* is not. Why does this matter? Is it a distinction without a difference? No. Even a mild B6 insufficiency has been shown to increase the risk of cardiovascular disease. Recently published epidemiological evidence shows how a reduction in dietary Vitamin B6 can lead to reduced concentrations of B6 in the blood and these studies seem to show that this reduced state can lead to an increase in cardiac risk. Strangely, no one agrees on how exactly B6 plays its important a role in contributing to heart health, but it seems very likely that it does.[5]

In fact, the presence of Vitamin B6 in a supplement makes folic acid (another B vitamin) able to do its job. In other words, B6 works synergistically with folic acid to help it stimulate revascularization of the arteries leading to the heart. For a long while, folic acid has received all the credit, but recent research seems to show that, without the presence of B6, folic acid would play no significant role in coronary revascularization. In support of this hypothesis, patients who had open-heart surgery or other significant cardiac surgeries, and did not have Vitamin B6 as part of the supplementation support, did not show vascular regrowth.[6]

B9 - Folic Acid/Folate

Folate, and it's sister term folic acid, come originally from the word "foliage" which is how you can remember which foods are good sources—it's in green leafy vegetables and beans! Folic acid has made a name for itself as a supplement used to prevent the risk of neural tube defects in the unborn child. But this B vitamin is not a one-trick pony. Folic acid supplementation has been used for decades to promote a drop in serum homocysteine levels with an eye toward achieving a lower incidence of heart disease.[7, 8] Elevated homocysteine levels are associated with greater risks of Alzheimer's onset and strokes.

In a 2012 meta-analysis (the mother of all scientific research), a team of researchers found that when all the evidence was gathered and analyzed together, it was possible to conclude that folic acid supplementation was useful in preventing future strokes.[9]

Folic acid also plays a remarkable, "almost magical" role in helping cure heart attacks and reduce the dysfunction that comes from ischemia (lack of oxygen) to the heart.[10] Supplementation with folic acid has been shown to reduce myocardial ischemia and decrease post-reperfusion injury.[11] The authors of a compelling editorial in the prestigious Circulation journal agree; they don't know exactly how folic acid works to heal damaged myocardial tissue, but they express confidence that it does. They make a strong case for continuing to pursue the reasons behind for the benefits of folic acid this way: "As the effects demonstrated here are so powerful, and as folic acid is highly affordable, further investigations are certainly warranted for both scientific and social causes."[10]

One word of caution, however... excessive intake of folic acid or folate can cause harm in many ways, so don't take more than the daily-recommended dose of 400 mcg. Even better, get it directly from vegetables!

B12

When people talk about the benefits of B vitamins, they often throw around concepts like elevated plasma homocysteine levels. So what are homocysteine, exactly, and why does it matter if the concentration of homocysteine in the blood is too high?

In short, homocysteine is an amino acid that is produced when proteins begin to breakdown. An elevated homocysteine level is considered potentially dangerous because homocysteine can damage arterial walls and lead to an increased risk of cardiac events, such as heart attacks. In India, many of the people suffer from low vitamin B12 status and high homocysteine levels, so they are the perfect population to investigate the effects of Vitamin B12 supplementation.[12] One such study investigated whether individuals could better reduce their homocysteine levels by eating lots of green leafy vegetables or by taking a Vitamin B12 supplement. The people who ate cooked green leafy vegetables showed no improvement in vitamin B12 levels, and their homocysteine levels failed to drop. Those people who took the supplements showed higher B12 levels and showed a significant drop in their total of high plasma homocysteine concentrations.

When scientists want to test for the benefits of Vitamin B supplementation, it is very useful to have a population of people who intentionally abstain from eating foods that are rich in Vitamin B12.[13] Vitamin B12 is found primarily in animal products, especially in red meat. Because vegetarians do not ingest meat, they are especially at a higher risk for Vitamin B12 deficiency. In a 2015 study, researchers looking at the effects of B12 supplementation drew a fascinating conclusion when looking at the classic vegetarian diet. They found that when compared with non-vegetarians, vegetarians have an improved cardiopulmonary risk "profile," but that this improvement was essentially wiped-out or negated because of the vegetarian's tendency towards B12 deficiency. Their scientific conclusion? Supplement with Vitamin B12.

Vitamin C

Vitamin C, commonly touted as being effective in fighting the common cold, is beneficial for so many other reasons. One of which is associated with hypertension. Studies have shown that for those with mild to moderate hypertension, this antioxidant vitamin is beneficial in reducing blood pressure readings.

Researchers cited that the notable effects were seen in those taking a dosage higher than that, which is considered to be a daily-recommended requirement. For those taking 500 milligrams of vitamin C, their blood pressure readings dropped by nearly 5 points. Researchers confirmed that this change was due to the natural diuretic effects of vitamin C, which removed sodium and water from the body.

Studies also concluded that vitamin C was effective in restoring the elasticity in blood vessel walls, aiding in the prevention of plaque formation.

When looking for a vitamin C supplement, choose one that is in combination with other vitamins and minerals, such as vitamin E, calcium, magnesium, and iron. While the daily recommended dosage of vitamin C is 60 milligrams, I recommend around 250 mg per day due to a general lack of the vitamin in the average diet. Amounts much higher than this are actually flushed out of the body without any effect. Note also that high blood sugar prevents the absorption of vitamin C.

{Vitamin C is effective in restoring the elasticity in blood vessel walls, aiding in the prevention of plaque formation.}

The best way to get your vitamin C is from fruits and vegetables! That way it comes with the rutin and bioflavanoids that allow it to be used as a whole food, and you avoid creating imbalances in your body that can happen when taking large amounts of an isolated vitamin.

Fat-Soluble Vitamins

Vitamin E

Vitamin E, a fat-soluble nutrient, is beneficial to protecting your body on a cellular level. This antioxidant can be found in many foods, such as olive oil, avocado, nuts, and green leafy vegetables. Like other antioxidant vitamins, such as vitamins A and C, vitamin E may play an important role in protecting your body from the cell damage caused by environmental free radicals (such as cigarette smoke and air pollution). It also has properties that are beneficial to hypertension, in that it is involved in the process of creating red blood cells, which helps to widen and prevent blood clotting in the vessels.

There has been some bad press about vitamin E in the research, and it's primarily because, instead of getting our nutrients from food, we take synthetic vitamins in large amounts and in isolation (meaning, without the other things that came with it in food), which is problematic and can cause some unintended side effects. This is especially true if you're on medication, as it can have adverse side effects. Vitamin E deficiency is rare in most individuals, so health experts agree that getting adequate amounts of vitamin E from natural food sources is best. But supplementation is another option, if you do not get adequate dietary amounts, or if you have certain health conditions and are not able to properly digest the fat required to properly absorb the nutrient.

It's important to note that vitamin E is actually made up of eight parts. So when choosing a vitamin E supplement, look for those listed as "mixed tocopherols" and not just "alpha-tocopherol" which is only one part of the eight.

Currently, the recommended daily allowance for natural vitamin E (d-alpha- tocopherol, d-beta-tocopherol) for adults age 14+ years is 15 mg (22.4 IU).

As always, it is important to talk to your doctor to decide what option is best for you prior to taking any dietary supplement.

The Blood Pressure Solution

Vitamin D3

Vitamin D has long been recognized for its beneficial role in bone health and immune system function, but many people don't know how important it is for maintaining a healthy blood pressure. Research indicates that vitamin D deficiency has been associated with a group of health problems, including insulin resistance, obesity, and hypertension. It is also a requirement for statin drugs to work effectively. Conversely, people with higher vitamin D intakes have lower average systolic blood pressure.

Vitamin D works to maintain a healthy blood pressure by increasing the absorption of calcium, which as we know plays an important role in cardiovascular health. Few people actually get enough vitamin D to reap the benefits that it offers.

You can get vitamin D in two ways: food (eggs, liver, butter, full-fat dairy, and some fish) or sun exposure. But most people only get around half of the 600 IU/day dietary intake recommended for people ages 1-70, and we generally don't spend enough time outside to make our own. Foods that are fortified with vitamin D, such as milk, yogurt, and cereal, usually have the less effective form—vitamin D2 (more on that in a minute).

> {Vitamin D works to maintain a healthy blood pressure by increasing the absorption of calcium, which plays an important role in cardiovascular health.}

If you're overweight, over 50, have diabetes or dark skin, or smoke, then you are at an even greater risk for vitamin D deficiency, because these factors can interfere with your ability to absorb dietary vitamin D or make your own vitamin D via sun exposure.

With all of these challenges to getting enough vitamin D, many people choose to use a dietary supplement that provides additional vitamin D. But not all types of supplemental vitamin D are created equal, and choosing the wrong kind can dramatically decrease the benefit of vitamin D supplementation.

The vitamin D found in supplements is D3, which is the form of D your body uses. D2 is found in small amounts in some plants and mushrooms, but it's very difficult to use in the human body and isn't typically sold as a supplement.

As with vitamins E and C, there can be unintended side effects to take large amounts of isolated vitamin D. The newest research is showing that vitamin D, taken without vitamins A or K2, can increase cardiovascular disease in levels over 45 mg/dL. So the best way to take it is either in combination with K2 or in a food form like cod liver oil, where it comes with vitamin A.

Vitamin K2

Vitamin K was first discovered in the 1930's. Scientists later recognized that there were two forms of Vitamin K known as K1 (phylloquinone) and K2 (menaquinone), but they didn't think that the two variations did different things. Today, we know better. While there is very little Vitamin K1 deficiency in the world, this is not true of Vitamin K2, and a deficit of

Vitamin K2 can have direct consequences on your heart and your bones. It's even important for promoting normal growth of babies in the womb, but today, we are going to focus on what Vitamin K2 does for the arteries and the heart.[14]

Vitamin K is a fat-soluble vitamin, and it works hand-in-hand with Vitamin D and Vitamin A, both also being fat-soluble. To simplify its role a bit, think about it this way: Vitamin K2 is responsible for activating a certain protein in the body. It acts like a catalyst (or a key in a lock). The presence of Vitamin K2 unlocks the matrix Gla protein (MGP), and this protein does a pretty amazing thing. It cleans excess calcium from inside your arteries and veins. It's acts a little like a custodian, cleaning the body's hemodynamic hallways of calcium debris. This singular role has a direct impact on heart health; if the arteries and veins are not routinely "maintained", plaque continues to layer, eventually occluding blood flow and leading to atherosclerosis. Since approximately one-fifth of all arterial plaque is actually excess calcium, Vitamin K2 gets to play a starring role in activating the protein that reduces this risk factor.[15]

It's interesting to watch the science catch up with science fiction on the role of K2. For a long while, the mainstream of researchers submitting to publications seemed to minimize any special role for Vitamin K2.

But in a 2015 article in the prestigious journal Atherosclerosis entitled, "Prevention of vasculopathy by vitamin K supplementation: Can we turn fiction into fact?" the authors discuss all the ways that Vitamin K2 does seem to play a very special role in heart health.[16] Some studies even suggest that Vitamin K2 can be more effective than Vitamin D2 at supporting healthy blood levels of calcium.[17] In fact, some physicians are calling it the new Vitamin D.[18]

The Blood Pressure Solution

Coenzyme Q10

Coenzyme Q10 (abbreviated as CoQ10) is a vitamin-like substance needed for proper cell function. Our bodies naturally produce CoQ10, and it is highly concentrated in several of our major organs, particularly the heart.

Author and nutrition expert Keri Glassman, confirms that researchers are excited to discover the importance of ubiquinol (the converted form of CoQ10) in maintaining cardiovascular health. According to Glassman, "CoQ10 and ubiquinol levels diminish with age . . . making cells more vulnerable to cell damage."[19] It is also depleted when people are taking a statin drug (often prescribed to lower cholesterol levels).

Scientists have found that CoQ10 has a positive effect in reducing cardiovascular complications, also indicating that those with previous heart-related conditions were deficient in this powerful antioxidant.

There has also been much interest in CoQ10 and how it affects blood pressure. Several studies indicate that those given CoQ10 supplements twice daily significantly reduced both systolic and diastolic blood pressures.

Some believe that adding a CoQ10 supplementation, in addition to effective diet and lifestyle changes, can reduce the need for prescribing multiple medications for those experiencing high blood pressure. Since CoQ10 is produced naturally in the human body, there are virtually no side effects resulting from supplementation of this antioxidant.

Omega-3s, 6s, and 7s

Omega-3 is a fatty acid that is not naturally produced by our bodies but is commonly found in fish like herring, salmon, trout, and tuna, and in smaller amounts in walnuts and chia seeds, as well. Flax oil also has Omega-3 fatty acids, but if someone has high insulin in their system from eating carbs, insulin prevents Omega-3's conversion into EPA and DHA. Another reason to stop eating sugar!

Fish oils have been the topic of much research regarding their effect in expanding the blood vessels, promoting cardiovascular health, reducing triglycerides, and lowering inflammation.

According to Dr. Jeremiah Stamler, professor emeritus of preventive medicine (Epidemiology) at Northwestern University in Chicago, "A large percentage of people between ages 20 and 60 have a rise in blood pressure, and by middle age, many have high blood pressure."[20] Based on the results of his study, he indicated that further research would be done in order to focus on the "dietary factors that may help prevent that rise, and Omega-3 fatty acids are a small, but important piece of the action," he said.[21]

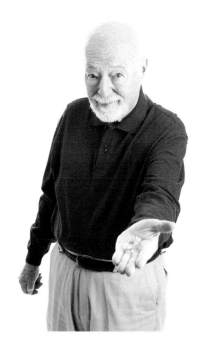

The study review results confirmed that there were significant reductions in both the systolic and diastolic blood

The Blood Pressure Solution

pressure. While there were insignificant results for those who did not have high blood pressure, the positive results achieved from the hypertensive group were encouraging.

This review confirmed previous conclusions about the positive effects of using Omega-3, as a supplement or via natural food sources (like fish, walnuts, or flax seed), for those with hypertension and potentially with those with other cardiovascular diseases.

However, for those who are currently taking prescribed antihypertensive medications, it is important to consult with your doctor prior to including any Omega-3 supplementation to make sure your blood pressure doesn't get too low.

Essential fatty acids are just that—fats that our body needs, but that we cannot produce ourselves. So this means we have to get them from foods. They get their description from their biochemical make-up, with the Omega-3's having a double bond *three* positions in from the end, and the Omega-6's having a double bond *six* positions in.

There are several different kinds of each of them, but they all start from the basic version and get converted from there. A couple of examples of Omega-3 fatty acids are DHA (docosahexaenoic acid) which is very important for good brain function, and another called EPA (icosapentaenoic acid) which helps to counter inflammation in the body. And Omega-6's are used in nearly every tissue in the body, especially during and after exercise to promote growth and limit cell damage from inflammation.

There are several places that modern humans have started to have problems with these fatty acids. The first place is

The Blood Pressure Solution

that all the converting doesn't happen, or doesn't happen as well, when people have elevated insulin levels from high sugar intake. This is the case for people who have trans-fats in their diets, or who are zinc, magnesium or B6 deficient, as well. The second problem starts with the change in the ratio of Omega-3's to Omega-6's.

Research says that we should have somewhere between a 1:1 and 1:4 ratio of Omega-6's to -3's. But these days, the average American has a typical ratio in excess of 10:1 and possibly as high as 30:1. There is also quite a bit of research showing that high Omega-6 intake causes a number of diseases like arthritis, inflammatory diseases (including heart disease), and cancer.[22, 23, 24]

At this point, you might be asking where we're getting all these Omega-6 oils. The most common place is the use of seed oils—corn, soybean, safflower, cottonseed, canola, and sunflower. The top two places these are found are in commercial salad dressings and in restaurant foods. The introduction of these oils changed the American diet, and the constant exhortation to stay away from saturated fats and use only liquid fats caused a shift in our bodies, and it was NOT in a good direction. Our bodies weren't meant to use all those liquid fats.

You might also be thinking that if the ratio is a bit off, then you should probably just take more Omega-3's. No, that won't fix the problem either—increasing that whole category of PUFA's (polyunsaturated fatty acids) will also cause health issues. Instead, reducing the amount of Omega-6 and sugar you consume are the two most important dietary things you can do for your health today! This looks like making your own salad dressing with real olive oil, and reducing how often you eat out. You should also increase your intake of other fats, like coconut oil, avocados, olive oil, etc.

There's another interesting fatty acid, which has started to gain some press. Omega-7's are in the same category as olive oil, as both are monounsaturated fats. Omega-7's help decrease insulin resistance, keeping our hearts and arteries healthy and our blood pressure normal. It lowers triglycerides and LDL, which translates into lowering blood sugar and insulin resistance (triglycerides) and reducing damage and stress on the body (LDL). It can be found in a balanced diet, but as you're beginning to realize, most of us don't have that!

Minerals

Potassium

Based on overall studies, researchers have found that "a reduced intake of sodium and increased intake of potassium could make an important contribution to the prevention of hypertension, especially in populations with elevated blood pressure."[25] Potassium appears to actually weaken the effects of excessive sodium intake.

Just like sodium, potassium is fundamental in maintaining adequate fluid and electrolyte balance. This essential macro mineral is significant to our brain, nerve, heart, and muscles performance, and for bone strength. "High potassium levels may act as a diuretic, causing sodium to be excreted,"[26] says Paul Whelton, MD. "Or potassium may dilate and relax the muscles in blood vessel walls."[27] Interestingly, this mineral has also been found to reduce the risk of stroke, yet Whelton continues, "most Americans get only half their recommended allowance."[28]

The current recommended amount of potassium needed for healthy adults is 4,700-mg/ day, which can be easily achieved by eating a balanced diet containing potassium-rich fruits and vegetables.

Currently, though, it's estimated that only 5% of Americans under the age of 50 are eating the recommended amount of vegetables, compared to only 10-25% over the age of 50. Which means that on average, most American adults do not consume enough potassium to reach the recommended amount necessary for adequate nutrition.

Magnesium

Magnesium is needed for over 300 biochemical processes within your body, and it should be no surprise that many of those processes will impact your blood pressure. In a study from the University of Hertfordshire, researchers found that "magnesium supplements may offer small but clinically significant reductions in blood pressure."[29] Combined studies further indicated that dietary supplementation of magnesium may have an effect in reducing blood pressure, particularly in higher dosages, according to the university's senior lecturer and registered nutritionist, Lindsy Kass.

As with potassium, doctors recommend making dietary modifications to include healthy fruits and vegetables in preference to supplementing your diet with extra magnesium. As always, this recommendation depends on the individual. If you cannot get the proper amount of magnesium through dietary means, supplementation is necessary.

The Blood Pressure Solution

Calcium

Calcium, the most abundant mineral in our bodies, is known to provide strength to our bones and teeth, but it also plays a lesser-known part as an electrolyte, important to several significant biological processes.

While less than 1% of our body's calcium reserve is needed to perform these functions, there has been much interest in its potential effect in lowering blood pressure.

Studies indicate that those who maintain a healthy, balanced diet, which includes foods containing calcium, magnesium and potassium, tend to avoid health issues associated with hypertension. Calcium helps healthy hearts contract, and calcium channel blockers lower blood pressure by weakening the heart's contractions. This process may be effective but a less desirable way to achieve healthy blood pressure control.

On the contrary, those who do not meet a sufficient intake of calcium in their diets tend to have higher blood pressure rates. Despite receiving mixed results, many researchers indicate that ongoing studies are warranted with regard to the positive effects that calcium may have in reducing blood pressure.

Selenium

Selenium, a trace mineral, is an essential micronutrient. As a component of an unusual group of amino acids, selenium works as an antioxidant, important to protecting our bodies on a cellular level.

Evidence suggests that selenium, shown to be effective in preventing inflammatory diseases, may also be effective in protecting against other conditions, such as atherosclerosis (vascular disease) and hypertension. Selenium is also very good at maintaining healthy thyroid metabolism, especially in the face of stress (cortisol).

Much research has been done on the effectiveness of selenium. The richest source of selenium is Brazil nuts, with 1 ounce containing 537 mcg of selenium, which is 767% of daily nutritional value. Mustard products are an excellent source of selenium (as well as calcium, potassium, and magnesium).

Natural Sea Salt

Unlike table salt, which is mined from the ground and typically referred to as mineral salt, natural sea salt is produced from the evaporation of seawater. Dating back to prehistoric times, this "good salt" has a unique flavor and can be used either in cooking or at the table.

While most brands of sea salt contain roughly the same amount of sodium as table salt, it also contains magnesium, potassium, and trace minerals that can help your body function better overall.

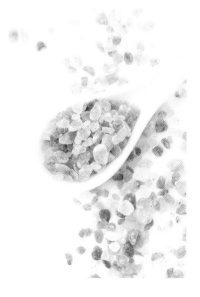

It's important to know when you go shopping that you might find a wide variety of options, and what you're

The Blood Pressure Solution

looking for is **_raw, unrefined_** sea salt. If it's white in color, or is made entirely of sodium chloride, then it's been refined or processed. You want one that has color (pink, gray, etc.), and that lists plenty of trace minerals.

Smart Supplementation

Anthocyanins

Anthocyanins are a powerful part of the group of flavonoids, notable for giving red, purple, and blue fruits and vegetables their colors. Many scientific studies have been performed to verify the positive effects that anthocyanins have in lowering blood pressure. Based on data collected, this flavonoid was found to be a major contributor to lowering a person's blood pressure, in comparison to other subclasses of flavonoids.

Experts agree that habitual consumption of foods containing this impressive flavonoid is therefore effective in providing a reduction in blood pressure levels because of its natural ability to increase nitric oxide.

Considering the encouraging data provided in these studies, consuming grapes, blueberries, pomegranate, strawberries, eggplant, and other similar food types, would be a safe and effective method for naturally reducing blood pressure levels.

Garlic

Overall, studies confirm that garlic is beneficial in lowering blood pressure, with most recent results indicating the success of using aged garlic extract as a safe and effective treatment.

Some have said that garlic is comparable in effectiveness to many antihypertensive medications such as beta-blocker, ACE inhibitors and ARBs (angiotensin II type 1 receptor antagonists). Garlic has been shown to have the ability to relax blood vessels and thin the blood, though this brings about concerns regarding the risk of potential interactions with certain drugs like Coumadin, which also have blood-thinning properties.

There has been much debate among experts regarding which specific form of garlic is most safe and effective in treating high cholesterol and blood pressure. Some believe that consuming raw garlic is most effective, due to diminishing benefits once cooked. Others indicate that while positive health benefits can be achieved, consuming large amounts of raw garlic for medicinal purposes may cause mild gastrointestinal side effects.

So, if you're wondering if there's any difference between raw and cooked garlic – yes, there actually is. It doesn't mean you have to eat it raw all the time, but a mix of raw and cooked will get you the most benefits. Let me explain.

Garlic, onions, shallots, and chives are all vegetables in a plant family that has a lot of sulfur. These sulfur chemicals are good for us and allow us to build our detoxifying proteins like glutathione. This is how we remove chemicals, drugs and heavy metals from our cells.

Garlic, however, is in a class of its own. It contains the parts to assemble a special sulfur molecule, allicin, which has made garlic famous for its miraculous benefits. The catch is that allicin is short lived and unstable.[30] It doesn't survive cooking, and it has to be frozen at -94 degrees F to be stored as an extract.[31] So how can we get it in us? The key is built into garlic itself. It contains a precursor, alliin, which is activated by an enzyme allicinase to make allicin. Crushing garlic turns the enzyme on and activates allicin. Eating raw—crushed or chewed—garlic delivers the allicin that lowers blood pressure. Allicin is sometimes listed in garlic supplements, but it is unlikely to still exist by the time you take it home. The key is, it can't be swallowed whole—it has to have the cells opened up to release the allinase enzyme, meaning it has to be cut up or broken up in some way.

Allicin reduces platelet stickiness and thins blood. Allicin blocks cholesterol-producing enzymes and lowers cholesterol. Allicin is probably the single most powerful prevention against cardiovascular disease. The absurdity of taking an aspirin a day becomes apparent when its risks of bleeding and modest benefits are compared to the immense benefits and lack of risk from garlic. Just note that garlic should be discontinued before surgeries due to its blood thinning effect.

Garlic can be easily added to a number of foods. If you like the taste of cooked garlic, use some of it in a recipe cooked, and add the rest of it raw, afterwards. Using a garlic press and adding some to any food after cooking will give you all of the

The Blood Pressure Solution

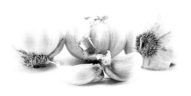

benefits. Adding raw garlic to salsa or hummus, refried beans or mashed cauliflower at serving, or mixing with a little butter to put on steak are all ways of using raw garlic. Add raw crushed garlic to pesto or guacamole. How much, you ask? A clove a day seems to be enough from what research has found.

Rutin

Rutin is a bioflavanoid discovered by Albert Szent-Gyorgyi, the same man who won the Nobel Prize in 1937 for discovering Vitamin C (ascorbic acid).[32] While studying the cure for scurvy, a bleeding disorder, another factor he called Vitamin P was found, which is now called rutin. Rutin stopped bleeding and edema by strengthening capillaries and reducing permeability (thus the 'P' in the original name of vitamin P). Ever since then, it has been known to help circulation, and recently more of its benefits have been discovered. Rutin stops an enzyme called protein disulfide isomerase (PDI). PDI is part of the clotting process, and rutin, a substance with no known toxicities at all, may be the safest substance to stop unwanted clots. Rutin safely blocks this enzyme outside of cells (preventing clots) while leaving it alone inside of cells (vital for making proteins).[33, 34]

This is a huge find in research, and is therefore a very hot topic among scientists. No drug can do the same thing without negative side effects.

Rutin is found in fruits and vegetables, like asparagus, apples, buckwheat and citrus fruits. It's usually found in foods containing vitamin C, so once again, it's all about eating a balanced diet!

Green or Oolong Tea

Tea is the most popular beverage in the world, but it's more than just liquid refreshment. It's also a great way to relax and unwind, and it's long been known to contain powerful antioxidants, especially if you pick the right type.

What makes the different kinds of tea different from each other is the way they're processed. If tealeaves aren't dried immediately after being picked, they will begin to wilt and oxidize, which alters the compounds inside. Black tea is allowed to wilt and oxidize fully before it is dried; green tea is dried immediately, and oolong tea is wilted, bruised/browned, and partially oxidized.

As it turns out, green, and oolong tea in particular, help to reduce the risk of hypertension.[35] Both contain less caffeine than black tea. Oolong contains catechins (an antioxidant), as well as calcium, potassium, selenium, and vitamins A, B, C, E, and K.

However, the findings reported that, despite these risk factors, the blood pressure readings for those who drank tea regularly were still lower than those of the non-tea drinkers. The study authors found that the most exciting results in their findings was the significant decrease in numbers of those who ultimately developed hypertension over the course of the study.

The researchers concluded that, "Compared with non-habitual tea drinkers, the risk of developing hypertension decreased by 46% for those who drank 120 to 599 milliliters per day, and was further reduced by 65% for those who drank 600 milliliters per day or more..."[36] So evidence indicates that by regularly consuming oolong tea, you are increasing your ability to naturally lower your blood pressure and reduce your risk of hypertension.

So cold or hot, oolong tea is a refreshing way to sit back and relax, and relieve some stress.

Green Tea Leaf Extract

There is no longer any doubt that the tea itself has extraordinary health benefits;[37] but what about an extract, made from the green tea leaves?

The savvy consumer should always question whether an extract or a pill could pack the same punch as the "thing" itself. So, when in doubt, look to the science. In 2012, a group of researchers asked a very similar question: can green tea extract provide the same benefits that the tea itself is known to provide? The scientists examined the supplement's effect on both obese and hypertensive patients, and their findings were amazing. In short, with daily supplementation, blood pressures went down, insulin resistances improved, inflammation decreased, LDL cholesterol levels went down (which was good) and HDL cholesterol levels went up (which was even better).[38]

But that's not all green tea extract has been shown to do. Another group of researchers asked similar questions, and got the same positive results as the group just mentioned, but they also asked several other questions.[39] First, they asked, what, if anything, could 3 months of daily tea supplementation do for antioxidant levels in the overweight or obese patient? Answer: increase antioxidant health. In other words, over a mere 90 day period, these individuals were able to convert their bodies into better fighters against cell damage brought on by stress, the environment, and bad habits, like smoking. Second, this team of researchers asked whether supplementation with green tea extract would produce any decrease in body mass index or waist circumference.

Well, it did. The patients' body masses went down and their waist sizes decreased. And lest you think such a finding is important only on a superficial level (improving how they "looked"), think again. Body mass index and waist circumference are excellent predictors of risk for cardiovascular disease. In fact, according to Mayo Clinic, individuals with apple-shaped bodies (those with larger waist circumferences) are much more likely to manifest the dreaded "metabolic syndrome" of diabetes and heart disease.[40]

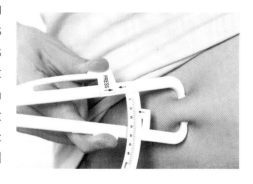

One last note. Whenever looking for the final word on scientific proof, it helps to look for something called a "systematic review" of the evidence. In a way, systematic reviews are "super studies" because they pull together all the existing studies, examine them, and state a conclusion about the combined weight of the evidence. I mention this here because the evidence supporting the usefulness of green leaf tea extract seems to have hit a tipping point. In 2015, researchers published a systematic review supporting the cardiovascular benefits of supplementation with green tea.[41]

Nitrates

Not to be confused with nitrites, which are substances often used in curing meat, nitrates come from dietary sources, like beets and leafy green vegetables, and are converted to nitric oxide within our system. The inner lining of our blood vessels, (called the endothelium) uses the nitric oxide as a vasodilator (widening the walls of blood vessels, increasing blood flow).

Research demonstrates that consuming foods rich in nitrates is effective in lowering blood pressure through a natural process of improving blood flow. Several studies have shown that beetroot juice, when consumed daily, can significantly reduce blood pressure levels in only twenty-four hours. Scientists believe that this is a result of the nitrates, which naturally occur in the beetroot juice.

Another study indicated that similar results were achieved in those given a nitrate supplement, though the study concluded that the supplement only reduced diastolic blood pressure and not systolic. Scientists agreed that additional research is warranted.

L-Arginine

L-Arginine is an amino acid naturally produced by the human body. Included in a team of other compounds, this amino acid participates in an important chemical reaction that produces nitric oxide.

Scientists have shown that vascular disease can be identified as a result of endothelial dysfunction, so researchers conclude that the presence of L-Arginine, as it relates to the production of nitric oxide, is a good indicator of healthy endothelial cells, thereby helping to decrease high blood pressure in clinical hypertensive patients.

Researchers suggest that while our bodies naturally produce this amino acid, individuals with poor diets or particular health issues would benefit by consuming foods containing arginine, including nuts, seeds, beef, pork, and poultry.

Capsaicin

Capsaicin, included as part of the capsaicinoids family, is responsible for the heat found in foods, such as cayenne and red peppers, and has been shown to be effective in reducing blood pressure and aiding overall heart health.

By stimulating specific neurons for releasing catecholamines, body temperature is increased, insulin sensitivity is improved, circulation is enhanced, and through this process, weight loss can occur. This process does use the B-adrenergic receptors, so a person on beta-blockers will not notice an effect.[42]

In addition to capsaicin, cayenne peppers are also high in vitamins A, B complex, and C, and they are rich in both calcium and potassium.

Hawthorn

Hawthorn, rich in flavonoids, is an herb that's been used successfully for centuries to treat cardiovascular conditions. It works by strengthening the heart and effectively aiding in blood circulation, and is the best herb to use for cardiovascular conditions of almost any kind. It's an extremely safe herb to use, as no herb-drug interactions have been reported or seen in research.

Kerry Bone, a world-renowned herbalist and chemist, with over 30 years experience, refers to hawthorn as "the most significant herb for ischemic and congestive heart disease . . . with considerable evidence and research to support its status."[43]

Quercetin and oligomeric procyanidins (OPCs), the same antioxidants found in grapes, are among the types of flavonoids that may be responsible for hawthorn's effectiveness, according to a study by University of Maryland University Medical Center.

According to Dr. James Meschino, recognized as a leading expert in nutrition, anti-aging, fitness and wellness, "Scientific and clinical investigations have shown that active constituents in hawthorn extract

{Hawthorn... "the most significant herb for ischemic and congestive heart disease..."}

can reduce high blood pressure via their influence on the angiotensin system, by acting as calcium channel blockers and by improving endothelial function. When taken with Coenzyme Q10, and in conjunction with other antihypertensive lifestyle measures, hawthorn supplementation is a key element in the natural management of mild to moderate high blood pressure."[44]

Olive Leaf Extract

The medicinal benefits of the leaves of the olive tree have been known since ancient times. Research studies are now finding that a supplement containing the ingredients found in olive leaf extract may be an effective therapy for many health conditions, including hypertension.

A study was conducted including twenty sets of identical twins, each considered to be "borderline" hypertensive. A thousand milligrams of olive leaf extract per day resulted in a significant reduction in both their overall blood pressure readings and their LDL cholesterol in only 8 weeks. The study participants who did not receive the supplements did not show a significant change in blood pressure.

Researchers believe that the relaxing effect to the walls of the arteries may have been a result of a combination of ingredients found in the olive leaf extract. Olive leaves contain secoiridoids, which include ligstroside, oleacein, and most importantly oleuropein. The high concentrations of oleuropein are what researchers believe are the most significant compound in reducing blood pressure readings.

The properties of oleuropein are shown to have a direct effect on the stiffness and resistance of arteries, aiding in improving the function of the inner lining of blood vessels and regulating blood pressure.

Based on the positive evidence from the study, health professionals recommend taking 500 mg of olive leaf extract, twice daily. Please do not stop taking any prescribed medications or take olive leaf supplements without prior consultation with your physician.

Apple Cider Vinegar

Apple cider vinegar, made from apple cider, is available in both a raw and processed form. Containing an array of vitamins and minerals, including potassium, sodium, magnesium, calcium, and phosphorous, many health experts recommend using the organic, unprocessed kind. This unfiltered form contains different compounds that many believe are responsible for its beneficial qualities as a natural treatment for a wide variety of conditions.

In addition to being effective at treating the symptoms of common colds, infections, and skin problems, apple cider vinegar is said to have positive effects for weight control and improving both cholesterol and blood pressure readings.

There are many testimonials touting the amazing results achieved, including one indicating a drop of 20 points in systolic blood pressure and 30 points in diastolic over period of about of three months.

The average recommended dosage is one glass of water daily, with about 2 tablespoons of raw, organic apple cider vinegar. It's important to note that due to the highly acidic nature of apple cider vinegar, it should always be diluted to

The Blood Pressure Solution

avoid the potential of eroding tooth enamel or burning your throat. Most who regularly use this treatment were honest in stating that the taste can be somewhat unpleasant, but the benefits far outweigh the offensive taste and smell.

To improve this problem, some suggested adding the apple cider vinegar to a small glass of juice initially, though this can greatly increase the sugar/carb content. Another recommendation was to add stevia, a natural sweetener, with 2 tablespoons of the vinegar to a glass of water, which also

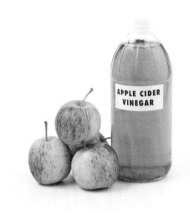

improved the taste. You can actually buy a drink like this at health food stores!

While there have been no reported harmful effects of using apple cider vinegar, it is always best to consult your physician prior to making changes to your dietary health plan.

Grape Seed Extract

Grape seed extract (GSE) is made from the seeds of red grapes, which are rich in vitamin E and linoleic acid. GSE, as well as all parts of red grapes (juice, skin and the seeds), is one of the most powerful sources of the flavonoid known as a proanthocyanidin, which is said to aid in reducing high blood pressure.

In a study including participants with metabolic syndrome who received 150 mg and 300 mg per day of GSE, lower blood pressure readings were achieved. Experts believe that the favorable result in improved blood pressure was due to the proanthocyanidin in the grape seed extract, which has a natural arterial relaxing effect.

Additional studies indicate that grape seed extract is beneficial to improving cardiovascular disease, hypertension, and blood cholesterol by supporting better blood flow.

Note that scientific evidence only supports the use of red grape seed extract (as opposed to white grapes). Including red grapes as a part of a heart-healthy diet is the best way to naturally receive the benefits of the antioxidants and flavonoids of this powerful fruit. Dietary GSE supplements are another alternative.

Pomegranate Fruit Extract

The pomegranate is one of the most clinically investigated fruits on the planet. Because of its long-standing history as a fruit favored by kings and gods (can we forget poor Persephone eating the pomegranate seeds and bringing the 4 seasons to mankind?), there has always been interest in whether or not the food stands up to its hype.

Pomegranate contains antioxidants with tough-to-pronounce names like ellagitannins. These antioxidants have been shown to help the body protect itself against free radicals, which damage the body at a cellular level. Because of this, the consumption of pomegranate juice has exploded in recent years. But what about the benefits of an alternative form of the juice – in other words, an extract? Recently, research teams tackled this question by investigating different preparations of extracts and they found that when patients consumed one or two capsules containing pomegranate extract, they demonstrated a change in their antioxidant activity.[45] The exciting part of these studies was the fact that the researchers didn't just look subjectively at the patients' quality of life. They measured how something at the chemical level (thiobarbituric acid reactive substances or TBARS, if you are dying to know!) reacted to the use of these extracts, and they saw a change. The levels of TBARS went down significantly (which, trust me, is what you want to happen); in other words, their antioxidant status improved.

Another group of researchers asked how the pomegranate stacked up against red wine or green tea infusions as a means to increase antioxidant health.[46] They already knew that both of these substances have been shown to help support both cardiopulmonary and metabolic health, so they wanted to know: was it possible for pomegranate to surpass their effects? Their results showed that yes, certain kinds of pomegranate preparations stimulated 3x more antioxidant activity than did either the red wine or green tea.

Interestingly, pomegranate consumption does more than just support the immune system; it also appears to help reduce clogging in the arteries, a condition referred to as atherosclerosis,[47] by reducing the serum ACE activity (a fancy way of saying that the levels of angiotensin converting enzyme (ACE) in the blood go down). Since a reduction in ACE activity has been shown to lead to less clogging in the arteries, a reduction of their levels would be an excellent start towards achieving greater heart-health.[48]

Amla Fruit Extract

The Indian gooseberry (known as Amla) is one of the world's super- fruits, and it's getting much more press recently. Used for centuries in many Asian countries, the western world is just catching on to its potential as an anti-inflammatory agent, which promotes better blood circulation. How can we know what consumption of this little berry's extract can do? One of the ways scientists know how to assess for heart health is through inspection of inflammation. One of the ways they know how much inflammation is present in the body is through measurement of something called C-reactive protein (CRP) levels.

Doctors can measure for your CRP levels through simple blood tests. In a way, they use such a test as a proxy, or a simple way to see if your body is in an increased state of inflammation. CRP levels are essentially a "marker" for inflammation: the more CRP, the more inflammation. And even though I'll bet you have never heard of a CRP blood test, they are just as predictive of cardiovascular risk as are cholesterol levels. Some studies even show CRP levels provide a greater predictive potential.[49] Amla has been shown to significantly decrease the blood levels of CRP.[50]

But that is not the whole picture for the lowly Amla berry. Amla appears to provide some coveted cholesterol benefits which normally only come about with extra trips to the gym (or good genes). The berry has been clinically shown to increase the body's levels of good cholesterol, known as HDL, while dropping the amount of "bad" cholesterol floating around in the blood stream.[50]

So what else can the Indian gooseberry do for you? It can support normal coagulation (clotting) of your blood and help keep your cholesterol and glucose levels in normal range.[51, 52, 53] It even helps regulate your blood pressure.[54] I'll bet that until now, you didn't even know its name!

Category 3: Reducing Body Fat

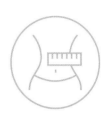

There is no doubt about the link between being overweight and high blood pressure. So this section describes the basics of how I've helped hundreds and hundreds of people lose weight without the needless suffering most diets impose. If you want more in-depth information on the subject of fat loss there's a resource at the end of this chapter that I highly recommend. But in this section, I want to share with you the basics—just enough for you to get started on the right foot.

Have a Big Reason Why

This is a critical component to breaking any old habit and starting a new one. You must know your own internal "reason why" losing weight is so important for you to achieve. Is it that you'd like to be healthy for your kids? Your grandkids? That you'd like to enjoy your old age without being on a cocktail of drugs?

Follow A "Real Food" Diet

The recommended foods listed earlier in this book are all considered "real foods" and will provide excellent nutritional value to your body. By eating only real foods, and staying away from things that come in a bag, a box, or can, many people notice an immediate 7–10 pound drop in body weight as their body sheds many of the toxins and excess water that they have been carrying around. To begin, just slowly start adding more "real foods" into your diet each week. At the same time you will start eliminating the overly processed and manufactured bad foods.

Pre-cook Your Food

One of the things that really help me stay on track is to do a little prep work, so that I'm not scrambling to find something to eat when I'm hungry. By pre-cooking my food for the week, I'm able to make much better decisions, and I'm less likely to go to a restaurant or grab a snack that comes in a plastic wrapper.

Limit Your Trips To Eat Out

Following on from the previous tip, I would highly suggest giving up eating out for a while, or at least limiting it to once, or maybe twice a month. Restaurants typically use way too much sodium, sugar, and processed oils, and have portions that are typically too big, encouraging us to overeat.

Drink Lots of Water

There is plenty of research that shows that thirst is often misinterpreted by the body as hunger. Often, drinking a full glass of water and waiting 10 minutes will take hunger pangs away. In addition, being dehydrated by as little as 2% can cause headaches, fatigue, and slow your metabolism.

The Blood Pressure Solution

Remember, your biochemistry relies on water for it to work. Without plenty of water, your cells do not function at optimum levels and this makes losing fat very hard.

Get Plenty of Sleep

The nighttime cycle of rest and regeneration is often overlooked as part of a sensible fat loss plan. However, I want you to know that it is essential. As your body rests and repairs the cellular damage from a normal day's activities, your body is also releasing powerful fat fighting hormones... as long as you are getting deep, restful sleep.

Measure Your Carb Consumption

The number one thing I recommend to friends and family who ask me how they can lose weight, is to drop their carbohydrate consumption down to under 100 grams of carbohydrates per day (to start). This will blunt the release of insulin into your system and help to keep fat burning going. If you go over 100 grams of carbohydrates and begin to inch up towards 150 grams of carbs per day, you will begin to notice fat starting to be deposited around your middle again. The release of insulin in your body not only causes fat to be stored in your body, but like I mentioned before, studies also clearly show its link to high blood pressure. The more added sugar you have in your diet (which spikes insulin in your body) the higher risk you have for hypertension.

Remember when I mentioned how counting calories is not considered the best way to lose weight? That's because they've realized that not all calories behave the same.

Where we got into trouble is when we looked at a gram of carbohydrates with its 4 calories per gram, and fat with its 9 calories per gram, then it looks like clearly you should cut fat out of your diet (which leads to eating high sugar/low fat, fake foods). But what they don't tell you is, that gram of carbohydrates came with the hormone insulin, and insulin not only stores extra calories as fat, it also prevents you from burning fat. You might be eating fat free cookies, but all that insulin is turning them into fat and keeping you from burning any of your extra fat.

Yes, you will lose weight if you eat less calories, but study upon study shows that's it's very hard to maintain that weight loss over time this way. It's not what I would recommend if you want to be healthy and lose weight in the long term.

Category 4: Exercise

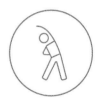

There are specific kinds of exercises that can be done at home, with no additional equipment other than your body weight. These exercises will dramatically improve your cardiovascular health. They can also trigger the release of beneficial hormones that will help you burn fat. In this section I'll share with you the type of exercises that work, without fancy equipment or doing "chronic cardio" on a treadmill!

In fact, this can be done in just 7–8 minutes per day! You may be wondering if exercising that little each day can have much of an impact on your health. Indeed it can if you keep the intensity level high enough.

The reason we are adding exercise to your health plan is to do the following:

1. Preserve muscle mass

2. Trigger release of fat burning hormones

3. Improve cardiovascular health

4. Increase metabolism

If you are very out of shape and have not done much, if any, physical exercise in the past several years, then the exercises shown below will be the perfect way to get back into working out. All of these exercises can be done at home and with no additional equipment. Instead, you'll use your own body weight to create resistance and begin to work your heart and cardiovascular system. It's designed to allow anyone to start moving and gain the confidence and strength needed to transition into more advanced workouts when you are ready.

You will set up your workouts based on a seven-day schedule. This allows you to keep a consistent schedule.

I can't overemphasize how important it is to work as fast as possible and make the exercise as intense as you can while still staying within the range of safety. The very best way to do this is to keep track of the time it takes you to complete the exercises below. Each time you perform them, try to beat your old time by a few seconds. If you continue to do this, you will essentially be working harder each time.

QUICK NOTE ON TERMINOLOGY:

In the descriptions I use the term 'round'. A round is simply one cycle through a set of exercises. If I was to say do two rounds of 10 push-ups and 10 air squats, then you would complete the exercises in this order:

Round 1:

- 10 push-ups 10 air squats

Round 2:

- 10 push-ups 10 air squats

OK, so let's dive into the Blood Pressure Solution workout. You can find the videos for these exercises inside your member's area.

Day One (typically a Sunday): this is a non-workout day, which allows your body to rest and recover.

Day Two:

- Warm Up: March in Place (4 minutes)

- 3 Rounds of:

  - 3 Get Ups!
  - 10 Air Punches

Get Ups! are simply lying down on the ground on your back fully extended, and then getting up into a standing position. Simple yet effective! Do this as quickly as possible.

Air Punches are simply standing with one foot in front of the other and then punching the air in front of you as if you were a boxer punching a bag. Alternate between right and left arms.

Day Three:

This is a non-workout day, but I want you to take a 10-minute walk to keep your muscles moving. This is a slow, leisurely walk.

Day Four:

- Warm Up: March in Place (4 minutes)
- 3 Rounds of:
  - 10 Wall Pushes
  - 10 Air Squats

A Wall Push is simply walking up to a wall, keeping your feet about 2' away from the wall, then leaning into the wall with your outstretched hands. Then you will do the same motion as if you were doing a push up, but in this case you are pushing against the wall.

An Air Squat mimics the movement you would do if you sat in a chair, but in this case there is no chair. You simply squat down as you would to sit in a chair, and then stand back up. Keep your feet pointing forward, and your back straight.

The Blood Pressure Solution

Day Five:

This is a non-workout day, but I want you to take a 10-minute walk to keep your muscles moving. This is a slow, leisurely walk.

Day Six:

- Warm Up: March In place (4 minutes)

- As many rounds as possible in 8 minutes:

    • 10 Wall Pushes
    • 10 Air Squats
    • 10 Air Punches

Day Seven:

This is a non-workout day, but I want you to take a 10-minute walk to keep your muscles moving. This is a slow, leisurely walk.

That's it! While this may look like a very simple exercise plan, you will find that by sticking with this very straightforward program you will begin to feel better, have more energy, and even start feeling stronger. Again, continually ramp up the intensity. For Days Two and Four, time yourself each week, and try to beat your personal best. For Day 6, try to do more rounds than you did last week. If you find that you have mastered these exercises and can blaze through them, you can begin to add hand weights to do the air squats and air punches. You can even get a weighted vest to wear that will quickly ramp up the intensity!

The best benefit, however, is that you will be conditioning your heart and blood vessels in a safe and effective way that will help to lower your overall blood pressure. Don't think that this simple exercise program is too easy for you! Try it out and you'll see that it works your whole body and that you will actually appreciate the rest days that are built in!

Category 5: Stress Reduction

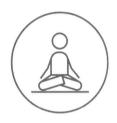

The reduction of stress plays a very important role in lowering blood pressure. Biologically, when we are under stress, our bodies react by releasing chemicals into our system in an effort to keep everything functioning properly. Not only are our minds and bodies working overtime, so are our major organs. Without proper diet and exercise, as well as adequate sleep, our systems will wear down and start to malfunction, causing all sorts of problems.

When you are stressed, your heart rate elevates, you tense up, and your biochemistry changes. Each of these things contributes to your blood pressure rising. In this section, I'll show you some extremely effective ways to lower your blood pressure with nothing more than your breathing, your mind, and a few simple techniques.

To begin, we can easily agree that we all experience some form of stress on a regular basis. It's practically unavoidable, right? Who hasn't ever wished to for the ability to just crawl into an imaginary hole of avoidance, desperately hoping that the momentary crisis will just magically go away? So it's fairly easy to recognize the outward symptoms of stress: avoidance, anxiety, anger, depression, headaches, and insomnia . . . the list goes on. But have you ever considered what's simultaneously happening to you on the inside?

To briefly explain the natural biological process, your body responds to stress by releasing a flood of hormones that trigger an increase in your heart rate and the narrowing of your blood vessels, which causes a temporary spike in your blood pressure levels.

In the heat of the moment, this short term elevation shouldn't put your body in any immediate danger, however science has proven that the long-term effects of this physical reaction to stress can put you at risk for developing serious health conditions—among them being hypertension.

While it has not been scientifically proven that stress actually causes high blood pressure, studies do indicate that there is indeed a link between blood pressure and stress. During a three-month study conducted by Dr. Randy Zusman (an expert in treating hypertensive patients), and in conjunction with Boston's Benson-Henry Institute for Mind Body Medicine, patients who were being treated with hypertension medications began participating in relaxation training.

Although somewhat skeptical of the effect that meditative actions would result in any significant results, Zusman was pleased to find encouraging results in about 40–60% of the patients involved in the study. "Their blood pressure dropped, and they dropped some of their medication. It was striking. It was statistically significant, but more important it was clinically significant to these people," he says.[55]

The Blood Pressure Solution

The doctor did further conclude that there is work involved in achieving these types of results. Learning to properly utilize the techniques, and becoming dedicated to following a daily meditation practice, is essential to achieving long-term results as indicated by the study patients who succeeded in lowering their blood pressure.

If you have been diagnosed with high blood pressure, or are concerned about its development, it's time to do something about it. Seriously, by dedicating yourself to taking command of your health and actively committing yourself to making permanent lifestyle changes, you can find yourself on the path of least resistance, steadily progressing toward better health.

How do you get the upper hand on stress? Realistically, it's your behavior (not the problem itself) that should be your first consideration. It's imperative that you grasp this truth: while you can't eliminate everything that causes complications in your life, you can (and **must**) take control of your reactions to them when they occur.

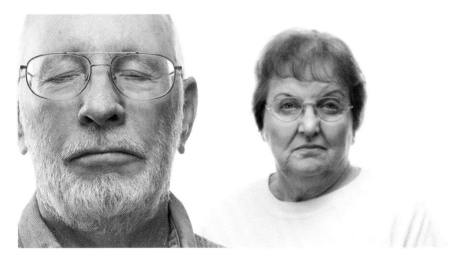

The Blood Pressure Solution

Mind-Body Interventions

Research has shown that a large majority of Americans are using complementary and alternative medicine treatments. This might involve meditation, relaxation and breathing techniques, biofeedback and autogenic training, acupuncture, and/or herbal remedies for the purpose of treating many health conditions. Below are brief explanations for a few of these stress-relieving techniques that are worthy of consideration.

Meditation

Meditation is a practice that is often misunderstood, for a variety of reasons. The most common assumptions are that meditation is just a type of religious practice, or else that it's another "new age trend." Neither are true. Meditation is focusing on one thing without the distraction of thinking. Can you imagine enjoying your dinner without thinking about what you had to do afterwards, or watching TV, or talking? Just enjoying the taste and sensation of your food? That's a version of meditation.

The intention for meditation is to *focus on something other than thinking.* We're all really good at thinking, usually too good, and this thinking becomes a stress when it's in the form of worry, when we can't be present with someone because of our thoughts, or when we can't shut it off before bed. If you can control this over-thinking even a little, it creates a "mini-vacation" for your mind, leading to health benefits that include not just reducing blood pressure, but improving digestion, sleep, and even slowing the aging process.

The Blood Pressure Solution

There are actually numerous types of meditational practices, which can range from a simple state of "daydreaming" to one that maintains a highly spiritual or religious focus. The techniques can vary by culture, and many are distinctive to each individual. But regardless of the specific technique, the basic premise of practicing any form of meditation is to focus your mind in a positive direction and improve your sense of well-being.

If you have never experienced meditation, just have an open mind and give it a try. Here is an easy form that I've taught my patients for years:

Either sit or lay down comfortably in a place that is quiet and where you won't be disturbed for 20 minutes or more. Close your eyes and notice how you're breathing. Are you breathing in "spikes", which people often do when they're stressed, or are you breathing in "circles", with one breath moving smoothly into the next? Just observe for a few breaths what is occurring.

Then, if you're not already there, bring your breathing to a "circle", with one breath moving smoothly into the next. Focus on the sound of your breath. What you'll notice is that, in about a half-second, you've started thinking again. When you notice that, just bring your focus back to the sound of your breath. Even if you have to do this 100 times, it's okay. You're training your brain to do something other than think!

Getting a brain pattern set takes about 2-3 weeks, so practice every day if you can, and don't get frustrated (since that's just another thought as well!). You'll notice that your ability to focus will start showing up in your daily life, from improved sleep to better concentration.

The Blood Pressure Solution

Breathing Properly

Related to the ability to relax is the ability to breathe properly.

"Just take a deep breath" is the advice often given to those experiencing moments of stress and anxiety. But does this really work? The answer is yes, but it must be done properly. Breathing exercises have been used for thousands of years as a way of calming your nerves and clearing your mind.

The most common type is referred to as "diaphragmatic breathing" (deep abdominal breathing). It is said that this technique can be used effectively to lessen anyone's tension; leaving you feeling relaxed as you control your internal rhythm. For those who are interested in using this technique for the purpose of lowering blood pressure, it offers excellent results when you are committed to practicing this method twice per day. Here are the basic steps:

1. Place one hand on your chest, the other on your abdomen. Inhale deeply, checking to ensure that the hand on your abdomen rises higher than that on your chest, to allow enough air into your lungs.

2. Calmly exhale, and begin inhaling, taking in a slow deep breath, and then hold it (but don't force it). To maintain control of your breath, count up to 7.

3. At the count of 8, begin to exhale slowly, until all of the air is released. Then contract your diaphragm muscles gently, and relax.

4. As when inhaling, be mindful of exhaling deeply and completely, but without forcing yourself.

5. Repeat this process 4 or 5 times. You should do 5 or 6 deep breaths, maintaining 5–6 breaths per minute.

A few practical tips when practicing breathing exercises...

•   Practice early in the morning, (or late in the evening) when your mind and body are relatively at ease, and the air is pure.

•   To achieve the best results, drink water approximately 30 minutes prior to beginning your exercises, and avoid practicing after consuming a meal.

•   Practice in an area that allows you to focus your attention strictly to the exercise, free of distraction.

Keep in mind the importance of making your breathing smooth and effortless. Start out slowly and take it easy as to avoid forcing yourself during your breathing exercises.

Biofeedback and Autogenic Training

Two stress relieving techniques that work well individually, or in combination, are biofeedback and autogenic training.

Biofeedback is a non-invasive technique that involves being connected to a machine that essentially trains you to do things such as consciously tightening or relaxing muscles in order to change your breathing patterns and can slow your heart rate. Based on the feedback you receive (via lights and sounds from the machine), you learn to be able to manage your stress by effectively controlling your muscle movements and breathing patterns.

Autogenic Training is a type of self-hypnosis. This technique is essentially learning how to reduce your tension by giving yourself silent instructions, such as "my head is clear and calm" or "my body is completely still and relaxed." While you can become very relaxed, you will still be aware of what's going on around you.

Much like meditation, these techniques used alone or in conjunction with one another allow you the freedom to control your thoughts and manage your stress in a safe and effective way.

Audio (Binaural Beats)

Your brainwaves and state of consciousness can be directly affected by certain auditory frequencies, varying from a state of high alert to one of deep sleep. At certain frequencies, the use of this auditory brain stimulation is said to induce a sense of calm and relaxation.

The method of using binaural beats works by introducing two specific auditory tones with a separate frequency per ear, heard through headphones. Your brainwaves then perceive the tonal variance and accommodate by producing a unifying third tone in order to naturally follow along with the beat.

To better explain, for example, if 200Hz were being played in your left ear, and 207Hz in your right ear, your brain perceives a tone of 7Hz. It has been proven that by using this technique consistently, you allow your brainwaves to synchronize and improve your thought processes.

The Blood Pressure Solution

Another great benefit of binaural beats (or tones) is that they cause your brain to start matching the frequency of the tone your brain perceives. In the previous example, where your brain would perceive a tone of 7Hz, your brainwaves would quickly start matching this frequency. The benefit to this is that certain brainwave frequencies have been identified that relate to specific relaxation states. For instance, brainwave frequencies of 4–8 Hz have been identified with deep meditative states—exactly what you need when you want to relax.

Brainwave Classification Chart

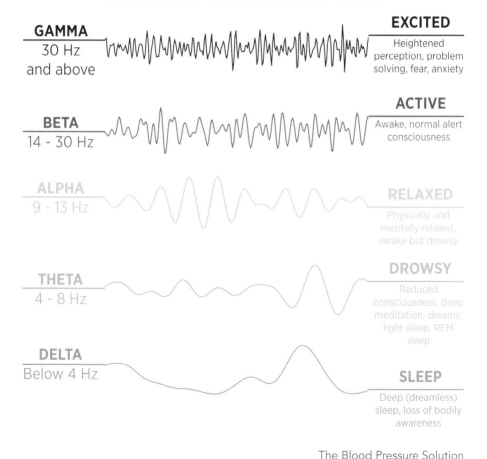

GAMMA
30 Hz and above

EXCITED
Heightened perception, problem solving, fear, anxiety

BETA
14 - 30 Hz

ACTIVE
Awake, normal alert consciousness

ALPHA
9 - 13 Hz

RELAXED
Physically and mentally relaxed, awake but drowsy

THETA
4 - 8 Hz

DROWSY
Reduced consciousness, deep meditation, dreams, light sleep, REM sleep

DELTA
Below 4 Hz

SLEEP
Deep (dreamless) sleep, loss of bodily awareness

The Blood Pressure Solution

While binaural beats have been proven to affect each listener in a mental and physical way, each individual hears the third "imaginary" tone differently.

If you have a smart phone, there are some free apps to try out binaural beats. Just go to your app store, search for "binaural", and try some out!

The use of binaural beats is not recommended for those who are prone to seizures, children, or while operating any type of machinery. As with any health condition, it is important to consult your physician prior to using this technique.

Acupuncture

Acupuncture is a practice used both in traditional Chinese medicine and by many practitioners of Western medicine. Though there is a variance in the purpose of practicing this alternative therapy, acupuncture has been shown to provide many health benefits. The technique involves stimulating the nerves in specific places of the body, using very fine needles to puncture the skin.

During this process, your body naturally releases certain chemicals and hormones in your body in order to allow the body to correct its imbalances.

Sometimes people get nervous at the thought of needles, but these are nothing like the hypodermics you are familiar with— these are so thin that they are practically the thickness of a hair. Many people are pleasantly surprised when they don't feel the needles and by how relaxed they can get, even at the first visit. This is one of the primary modalities we use in my office, because it's so effective.

By correcting the root problems associated with hypertension, such as the condition of your nervous system, blood vessels, and kidneys, acupuncture can have a positive effect in lowering blood pressure.

Acupuncture can be a safe, low-risk option for treating the symptoms associated with high blood pressure, but should only be done only by a professionally licensed practitioner.

Sleep

Just like many of us reaching the end of a long day, you're likely desperate to bring that day to an end, and just go to sleep. But how often do you find yourself tossing and turning in a constant struggle to get some shut-eye? Poor sleep not only causes stress and understandable fatigue, but it can lead to some serious health complications that should not be ignored, particularly if you have high blood pressure.

There have been many studies showing that insomnia, or a lack of sufficient sleep, can be directly related to having high blood pressure. If you are among the millions who have been diagnosed with hypertension, there is even more bad news. Researchers are now discovering that you are likely to double your risk of developing a resistance case of hypertension if you aren't getting the rest you need.

So what does this mean? Bottom line: you could be facing the possibility of being prescribed at least three hypertension medications, which unfortunately may prove to be ineffective in maintaining healthy blood pressure. Additionally, you're facing the challenge of a greater risk of developing any number of other associated diseases, which isn't encouraging.

The Blood Pressure Solution

Let's take a look at how a lack of sleep plays a role in your body's processes.

For illustration purposes, let's say you find that, over the years, you've put on a few unwanted pounds. As you've aged and your metabolism is beginning to slow down, your weight is steadily increasing. Without having made any positive improvements in your diet and exercise routine, you've reached the point of being considered overweight or obese. By now, in doing absolutely nothing, you've already placed yourself at a higher risk of developing any number of diseases.

Since we're focusing on things that disturb your resting period, let's start with the example of sleep apnea. This is a condition in which you wake up gasping for air several times during the course of the night, which causes disruption in your sleep patterns. Now let's say that this lack of quality sleep then turns into eating "fast food" because you're too tired to attempt to prepare anything healthy. As the pounds are adding up, so is your risk for developing hypertension, diabetes, and kidney problems (assuming you don't have it already).

Without any major modifications in your lifestyle, you'll still find that you're not getting enough rest, because the stress of dealing with these conditions is keeping you up all night!

This frustrating cycle of "cause and effect" symptoms is a clear indicator that your biological system is all out of whack. If you're not taking these symptoms seriously, you're just pushing yourself closer toward coronary heart disease, stroke, or worse... death.

Not getting enough sleep can lead to some pretty scary stuff, if you're not careful. But by making some adjustments in your sleeping habits, in addition to other necessary lifestyle changes, you can get one step closer to lowering your blood pressure, and improving your health.

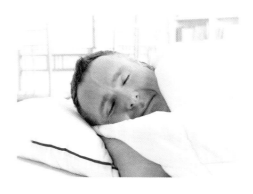

Tips for getting some quality sleep:

- **Sleep according to schedule**: go to bed and wake up at the same time, every single day (Yes, including on the weekends). This consistency promotes better sleep at night.

- **Stay calm:** if you find yourself tossing and turning, get up and do something relaxing. Try the meditation technique I taught you earlier. It can be very helpful for calming down your mind to sleep.

- **Don't go to bed hungry... or full:** avoid the distraction of gastrointestinal discomfort.

- **Limit your liquids:** try to prevent those late night trips to the restroom.

- **Avoid** alcohol, nicotine, and caffeine, each of which has stimulating effects.

- **Turn off the screens:** Computers, tablets, e-readers, phones, and TV's all of these lighted screens can change your brain patterns when watching them at night. Turn them off a minimum of 30 minutes before going to bed, and read a book instead.

- **Create a bedtime ritual:** take a shower, listen to soothing music, read a book, meditate... make relaxing a nightly habit to tell your body that it's time to go to sleep

- **Create a comfort zone:** create an environment that is comfortable for sleeping—not too hot, not too cold, not too bright, but just right. Be sure that when you are going to sleep, your bed is comfy cozy.

- **Try a catnap:** avoid taking a long nap during the day, which interrupts your normal sleep cycle. If you feel that you need to rest during the day, keep it quick. Enjoy an afternoon nap, but only for 10–30 minutes.

- **Get physical:** maintain a regular exercise schedule, and plan your physical activity well before bedtime to avoid being too energized to sleep.

- **Get a grip:** prioritize and organize to manage your daily stressors. Be intentional about creating time for yourself to unwind, using whatever relaxation techniques necessary to calm your mind, and relieve your stress.

- **Pick up the phone:** if your inability to sleep is causing disruption that is affecting your health, call your doctor. Seek the advice of a professional to diagnose and treat any potential disorders that may be keeping you up at night.

The Blood Pressure Solution

In the end, when facing the challenges of managing hypertension, and reducing your risk of developing other associated diseases, it's imperative to give equal consideration to spending time relaxing. Your body requires rest in order to rejuvenate and to function properly. As with anything, there isn't a "one-size-fits-all" method of relaxation. So feel free to try different techniques and see what suits you.

Either way, your end goal is always that of relieving your mind of anxiety.

Category 6: Eliminating Toxins

As you know, the things we put into our body can either help us or harm us. And two of the major offenders when it comes to hypertension are smoking and alcohol use.

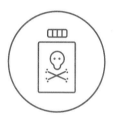

Smoking

One of the many, many harmful effects of smoking is that it raises your blood pressure. With each inhalation, the toxic nicotine constricts your arteries, permitting less room for blood to flow through and having the obvious impact. Having watched several family members struggle with smoking addiction, I'm sensitive to those that want to quit but are having trouble.

Just imagine with me for a moment:

If you quit smoking right now, twenty minutes later your heart rate slows down to a calm, steady beat, lowering your blood pressure.

Eight to twelve hours later, the dangerous levels of carbon monoxide in your blood have now dropped to a normal level. You may start to feel relief from any flu-like symptoms—from everyday fatigue to headaches, sleepiness, and nausea, all of which could have resulted from the effects of carbon monoxide.

Two days later, your heart attack risk is lower and continues to decline over the next three months. You'll suddenly notice that you don't need as much salt on your food (thanks to a return in the sensitivity of your taste buds), and the air smells fresh (now that your sense of smell has returned).

Three days later you might feel like going for a jog—because your energy is going to skyrocket.

After the first month, you have fewer instances of that annoying, hacking, smoker's cough because your bronchial tubes are on the mend. Whenever your bronchial tubes are irritated, they produce excess mucus. Eliminate the cigarettes, and you can say goodbye to the nagging feeling of having to constantly clear your throat.

A few months later, you'll be taking the stairs without gasping for a breath. As you get your body moving, your circulation will naturally improve, recovering from the effects of constricted blood vessels. Just one cigarette reduces the blood flow throughout your body for an hour.

The health improvements continue long after you quit smoking. Your gift at the first anniversary of quitting is that your risk of coronary heart disease becomes half that of what you risked as a smoker.

Here's another benefit: You'll keep aging signs at bay. The mouth suction that you use to puff on the cigarette is terrible for producing or deepening wrinkles. When you stop smoking, you give those facial muscles a well-deserved rest.

Make it to your fifth year smoke-free, and your risk of stroke is the same as that of a non-smoker. In ten years, your lungs become stronger, and your chances of dying from lung cancer are only half as great as if you had continued to smoke.

OTHER RISKS DECREASE WHEN YOU END YOUR SMOKING HABITS.

Here are a few more to consider:

- Cancer
- Cardiovascular Disease
- Impotence
- Infertility
- Macular Degeneration
- Periodontal Disease
- Ulcers

Alcohol Consumption

If you consume more than two drinks per day (for men) or one drink per day (for women) then you are putting yourself at a much greater risk for high blood pressure.

There are two reasons for that:

First is weight gain. Whether your alcohol contains little sugar content (dry wine, for example), or a high sugar content that comes with an insulin reaction (margarita, anyone?), both have calories. And those calories add up to the weight gain that negatively impacts your blood pressure. It's a good idea to limit your alcohol if you'd like to lower your blood pressure.

Second, alcohol overworks your liver. When the body detects alcohol in your system it treats it much like it would any toxin. It begins an all-hands-on-deck process to get it out of your body as fast as possible.

However, this is not as easy as it sounds. Alcohol must be broken down in your liver through a process called oxidation. Once the initial stages of oxidation occur, about 10% of the remaining by-products are eliminated from your body through your breath or your urine. The remaining 90% of the alcohol by-products are further broken down in the liver and turned into acetaldehyde.

The problem is that this process of breaking down alcohol takes a very long time—a full hour per average shot, 5-ounce glass of wine, or 12-ounce beer (or more, if that drink has a higher alcohol content). While your kidneys are busy using its resources to get rid of the alcohol, it neglects a few very important functions like the production of renin and

The Blood Pressure Solution

angiotensin, two proteins that are essential to keeping your blood pressure within normal ranges.

So although red wine can actually help reduce blood pressure (because of the presence of anthocyanins, which we discussed in the section on vitamins and minerals earlier in this chapter), overconsumption of any kind of alcohol has a negative effect.

CHAPTER 6

The Blood Pressure Solution: Implementation Plan

This book has given you a wealth of information about how to naturally lower your blood pressure. However, from this point forward I want you to think of it as a reference guide, rather than a list of things you **must** do right now.

Why? Because there is so much information here that you could easily get overwhelmed. But here's a very important tip:

No one can implement everything in this book on day one!

So relax! I'll show you my top recommendations for your first thirty days, which will help build an easy-to-follow daily plan, and give you a framework for monitoring your results. But don't feel like you have to do all of it at once—just put in what you can, and continue to monitor your progress week to week.

Small Changes Make a BIG Difference

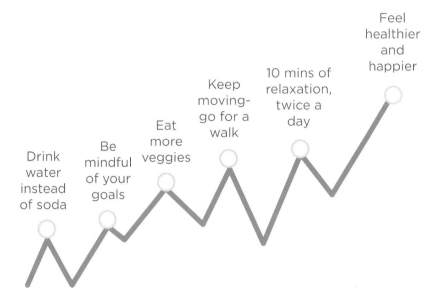

Then, when you are ready to try something new, just pick up this guide and read about the next supplement, exercise, meditation technique, or food that you want to include in your new healthy lifestyle.

How To Create Your Personalized Plan

We will be using a common feedback mechanism of *Implementing, Monitoring, and Adjusting* to make sure you are continually moving toward normal blood pressure ranges. Applied on a seven-day weekly schedule, this simple framework will create a predictable pattern for you that will allow any changes to your diet, exercise, or supplements to show their effect by the time you take new measurements at the end of the week.

With that in mind, get a notebook or a calendar that you can use to fill in the information for each of the five major categories you will be working on each day. Set aside a specific time once per week to do the bulk of the work— identifying which of the five categories you're going to work on, assessing the previous week's results, planning your meals, taking your measurements, creating a daily plan, etc. It shouldn't take very long. Then repeat the process next week.

1. Take Your Measurements

It has long been known that if you want to improve some aspect of a person's performance, you simply begin measuring their results. The same idea applies to your health. The very act of measuring your blood pressure, weight, and body fat percentage will help you become more aware of what you are eating. In addition, the data from each measurement will give us valuable data points so that we can monitor the impact of your new choices. If your measurements are not improving, then we know that we need to make adjustments. If they are improving, we know we are on the right track.

Recommendation: Each Sunday take three measurements:

1. **Body weight.** As you know, losing weight is a very effective way to drop your blood pressure.

2. **Body fat percentage.** This is also an indicator of obesity, and will help us see the progress you are making. To calculate your body fat percentage, just log in to the BloodPressureSolution.com Member's Area, click on the TOOLS tab, then type in your body weight and a

few simple measurements, and it will approximately calculate it for you.

3. **Blood pressure.** Obviously, this is the one we're trying to affect, so this is the one we need to be keeping the strongest eye on.

Every week, mark the results down in a notebook or a spreadsheet.

We also have a Blood Pressure Tracker tool in the Member's Area. With these three measurements, you will clearly be able to see any progress or regression you make each week, and easily identify if/when any adjustments are needed.

2. Assemble Your Meal Plan

The biggest leverage point we have to attack high blood pressure is your diet. By helping you transition to a lower carb, higher fat, medium protein diet that removes most processed sodium, you will begin to feel better within days, and your blood pressure will come down.

Recommendation: To create your ideal diet I want you to start with the included meal plans that came as part of

For more information about how you can receive hassle-free, weekly meal planning guides—complete with recipes that meet our special macrontrient ratios, and including the shopping lists, go to: perfectmealplans.com your purchase. Each of these recipes has been created to be very high in the foods that will naturally lower your blood pressure.

In addition to adding in these beneficial foods, one of the most important things you can do is to reduce your sodium intake by minimizing any and all processed foods.

3. Plan Your Exercise

Having a strong cardiovascular system is one of the smartest things you can do to help naturally lower your blood pressure. We will use short, but intense, exercises to stimulate your cardiovascular system and help improve its capacity. In addition, the type of exercise you will be doing has been shown to release certain beneficial hormones that help with fat loss and also muscle retention.

Recommendation: Refer to Chapter 5 of this book and follow the exercise plan as outlined, day by day. This exercise plan was created to trigger the release of fat burning hormones (and other beneficial hormones that will aid in fat loss), and is proven highly effective. It only takes 7–8 minutes a day, as well.

4. Take Time To Relax

We all live in a more stressful time now than our ancestors did, so want to incorporate two planned relaxation sessions per day. This is crucial, and I can tell you from my own experience, and the experience of my patients, that relaxation has a bigger effect than you can realize. These times of slowing down for a few minutes each day really do have a big impact on your overall stress level, which we know contributes directly to your blood pressure readings.

Recommendation: Each day set aside two 10-minute periods of time when you will utilize one of the relaxation methods presented in this book. I suggest taking 10 minutes in the 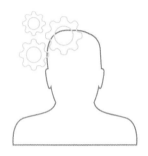 morning (shortly after you get up), and also one just prior to going to bed in the evening. Pick two of the methods presented in the section on Relaxation. You don't have to be a hard-core meditator to do this. Some of my best, and most relaxing, times were simply laying down, listening to calming music, and doing deep breathing. It is amazing how rejuvenating these simple actions can be—on both your mental outlook and your internal health!

5. Supercharging Your Results With Supplements

As much as we would all like to believe that our modern food supply could give us all the nutrition we need, the sad fact is that due to the customary processing of much of our food supply, many of the beneficial nutrients have been removed. To overcome this modern dilemma, many of us will need to supplement our diet with external sources. The following supplements are my top choices, and support the process of naturally lowering your blood pressure.

Super Supplement #1: Omega-3s

Super Supplement #2: Magnesium

Super Supplement #3: Potassium

Super Supplement #4: Hawthorn

Super Supplement #5: Grape Seed Extract

Super Supplement #6: D3

Super Supplement #7: Co-Enzyme Q10

Super Supplement #8: Nitrates

Make sure to visit the supplement section in your Member's Area for additional information on these supplements and how to order them.

Small Changes Make a Big Difference

As I said at the beginning of this chapter, no one can do everything all at once. Between the morning donuts your co-workers bring into the office, and the invitations to skip your scheduled workout and go to the bar instead... and between the new must-watch show on Netflix and your cell phone constantly dinging at you while you're trying to relax... and between the Thanksgiving dinner and even the candy bars at every single checkout counter in America, it's easy to feel like the entire world is conspiring against you. Life happens, and we all have to consider the choices we make in everyday circumstances.

The Blood Pressure Solution

But I want you to realize that even a small change can make a big difference. If the only thing you do after reading this book is replace conventional salad dressings with olive oil and vinegar, this alone could add five years to your life—no joke. I've known many people who've lost 10 lbs. just by cutting out soft drinks—which reduces blood pressure by 5-10 points, which in turn reduces the risk of stroke by 34% and the risk of a heart attack by 21%, especially if your waist size shrinks.

The *last* thing I'd ever want is for this to be a temporary phase for you—just another diet plan that you follow for three weeks before giving up. So pick a change. Just one. Make it something small, that'll be easy for you to do, so you can start off with a win. And watch that small change make a big difference!

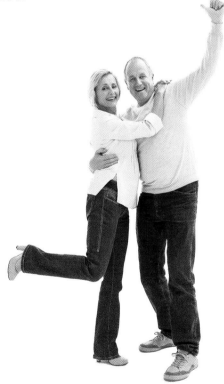

Conclusion

I spent years making a lot of the same mistakes you and many other people have made, and even years more putting together all of this information in a way that made sense both to me and to my patients. I had to redo all my thinking about fats, and about "good carbs", and how exercise fits into this. I had to figure out where patients succeeded and where others didn't, and how to adjust my recommendations. After years of doing this, the medical establishment is finally starting to catch up, using many of the same recommendations.

Instead of waiting for them (since, like I said, research is often 10 years ahead of standard medical advice), I'm just going to give this information to you directly, so that you can take control of your own health and get yourself back on the path to feeling good and being well!

Thank you for wanting to take back your health and for allowing me to be a part of that journey.

References

Introduction

1. (March 20, 2013). "High Blood Pressure Facts." *Centers for Disease Control and Prevention. USA.gov.* Retrieved from http://www.cdc.gov/bloodpressure/facts.htm.

2. (March 19, 2013). "Heart Disease Facts." *Centers for Disease Control and Prevention. USA.gov.* Retrieved from http://www.cdc.gov/heartdisease/facts.htm.

Chapter 1

1. (April 23, 2013). "High Blood Pressure." *MedlinePlus, U.S. National Library of Medicine.* Retrieved from http:// www.nlm.nih.gov/medlineplus/highbloodpressure.html.

2. (Mar 1, 2013). "What is High Blood Pressure?" *American Heart Association.* Retrieved from http://www.heart.org/HEARTORG/Conditions/HighBloodPressure /AboutHighBloodPressure/What-is-High-Blood- Pressure_UCM _ 301759_Article.jsp.

3. Bakris, George L., MD (March 2013). "High Blood Pressure." *The Merck Manual, Home Health Handbook. Merck Sharp & Dohme Corp, Merck & Co., Inc.* Retrieved from http://www. merckmanuals.com/home/heart_and_blood_vessel _disorders/high_blood_pressure/high_blood_pressure.html.

4. Hayward, Rodney A., and Harlan M. Krumholz. "Three reasons to abandon low-density lipoprotein targets an open letter to the Adult Treatment Panel IV of the National Institutes of Health." *Circulation: Cardiovascular Quality and Outcomes* 5.1 (2012): 2-5.

Chapter 2

1. Virmani, Renu, et al. (2002). "Pathology of the unstable plaque." *Progress in cardiovascular diseases* 44.5: 349-356.

2. (Jan. 21, 2011). "High blood pressure dangers: Hypertension's effect on your body." *Mayo Clinic. Mayo Foundation for Medical Education and Research.* Retrieved from http://www.mayoclinic. com/health/high-blood-pressure/HI00062.

3. (October 31, 2012). "High Blood Pressure Damages the Brain in Early Middle Age." *UC Davis Health System*. Retrieved from http://www.ucdmc.ucdavis.edu/publish/news/newsroom/7118.

Chapter 3

1. (March 26, 2013). "Black men continue to lead in hypertension statistics." *NewsUSA*. Retrieved from http:// www.stltoday. com/ lifestyles/health-med-fit/golden-age/black-men-continue-to -lead-in-hypertension-statis-tics/ article_99804a15-b5e8-5456 -a9b2-35a598263397.html.

2. Mattes, R. D., and D. Donnelly. "Relative contributions of dietary sodium sources." *Journal of the American College of Nutrition* 10.4 (1991): 383-393.

3. Adrogué, Horacio J., and Nicolaos E. Madias (2007). "Sodium and potassium in the pathogenesis of hypertension." New England Journal of Medicine 356.19: 1966-1978.

4. Graudal NA, Galloe AM, Garred P (1998). "Effects of sodium restriction on blood pressure, renin, aldosterone, catecholamines, cholesterols, and triglyceride: a meta-analysis." *Journal of the American Medical Association* 279.13: 83–91.

5. Garg, Rajesh, et al (2011). "Low-salt diet increases insulin resistance in healthy subjects." *Metabolism* 60.7: 965-68.

6. Stolarz-Skrzypek, Katarzyna, et al. (2011). "Fatal and nonfatal outcomes, incidence of hypertension, and blood pressure changes in relation to urinary sodium excretion." *Journal of the American Medical Association* 305.17: 1777-1785.

7. Ferrannini, Ele (2004). "Insulin and Blood Pressure: Connected on a Circumference?" *Hypertension* 45.3: 347-48.

8. Taubes, Gary (1998). "Three decades of controversy over the putative benefits of salt reduction show how the demands of good science clash with the pressures of public health policy." *Science* 28.1: 898-907.

9. "Taking Low-Salt Advice With A Grain Of You-Know-What" (May 26, 2016). *New York Times.* Retrieved from http://www.nytimes.com/2016/05/27/upshot/take-low-salt-advice-with-a-grain-of-you-know-what.html?_r=0

10. "Dash of Salt Does No Harm. Extremes Are the Enemy." (August 25, 2014). *New York Times.* Retrieved from http://www.nytimes.com/2014/08/26/upshot/dash-of-salt-does-no-harm-extremes-are-the-enemy.html?_r=0

11. Mente, Andrew, et al (2016). "Associations of urinary sodium excretion with cardiovascular events in individuals with and without hypertension: a pooled analysis of data from four studies." *The Lancet.*

12. Strom, Brian L., Ann L. Yaktine, and Maria Oria, eds (2013). "Sodium intake in populations: assessment of evidence." *National Academies Press.*

13. Sullivan, JM (1991). "Salt sensitivity. Definition, conception, methodology, and long-term issues." *Hypertension* 17.1:61-8.

14. Sanada, Hironobu, John E. Jones, and Pedro A. Jose (2011). "Genetics of salt-sensitive hypertension." *Current Hypertension Reports* 13.1: 55-66.

15. Svetkey L, Chen Y, McKeown S, et al (1997). "Preliminary evidence of linkage of salt sensitivity in Black Americans at the ß2 adrenergic receptor locus." *Hypertension* 29.4: 918-22.

16. Cooper, R, C. Rotimin, and S. Ataman, et al (1997). "The prevalence of hypertension in seven populations of West African origin." *American Journal of Public Health* 87:160-68.

17. Peters, Rosalind M., and John M. Flack (2000). "Salt sensitivity and hypertension in African Americans: implications for cardiovascular nurses." *Progress in Cardiovascular Nursing* 15.4: 138-144.

18. Weinberger, M., U. Wagner, and N. Fineberg (1993). "The blood pressure effects of calcium supplementation in humans of known sodium responsiveness." *Hypertension* 6.7: 99-805.

19. Weinberger, M., J. Miller, and F. Luft, et al (1968). "Definitions and characteristics of sodium sensitivity and blood pressure resistance." *Hypertension* 8.suppl II: II127-II134.

The Blood Pressure Solution

20. DiNicolantonio, James J., and Sean C. Lucan (2014). "The wrong white crystals: not salt but sugar as aetiological in hypertension and cardiometabolic disease." *Open Heart* 1.1: e000167.

21. Graudal, N.A., A.M. Galloe, and P. Garred (1998). "Effects of sodium restriction on blood pressure, renin, aldosterone, catecholamines, cholesterols, and triglyceride: a meta-analysis." *Journal of the American Medical Association* 279.13: 83–91.

22. O'Donnell, M, A. Mente, and S. Rangarajan, et al (2014). "Urinary sodium and potassium excretion, mortality, and cardiovascular events." *New England Journal of Medicine* 371.6: 12–23.

23. O'Donnell MJ,Yusuf S,Mente A, et al (2011). "Urinary sodium and potassium excretion and risk of cardiovascular events. *Journal of the American Medical Association* 306.22: 29–38.

24. Vasdev S, and J. Stuckless (2010). "Role of methylglyoxal in essential hypertension." *International Journal of Angiology* 19.e: 58–65.

25. Pollare T, H. Lithell, and C. Berne (1990). "Insulin resistance is a characteristic feature of primary hypertension independent of obesity." *Metabolism* 39.1: 67–74.

26. Brown, IJ, J. Stamler, and L.Van Horn, et al (2011). "Sugar-sweetened beverage, sugar intake of individuals, and their blood pressure: international study of macro/micronutrients and blood pressure." *Hypertension* 57: 695–701.

27. Hwang I.S., H. Ho, and B.B. Hoffman, et al (1987). "Fructose-induced insulin resistance and hypertension in rats." *Hypertension* 10: 512–16.

28. Preuss, H.G., and R.D. Fournier (1982). "Effects of sucrose ingestion on blood pressure." *Life Sciences* 30.8: 79–86.

29. Young, J.B., and L. Landsberg (1981). "Effect of oral sucrose on blood pressure in the spontaneously hypertensive rats." *Metabolism* 30: 421–4.

30. Centers for Disease Control and Prevention. "Leading Causes of Death." Retrieved from http://www.cdc.gov/nchs/fastats/leading-causes-of-death.htm.

31. American Diabetes Association. "Overall Numbers, Diabetes and Prediabetes." *Statistics About Diabetes.* Retreived from http://www.diabetes.org/diabetes-basics/statistics/.

32. Lustig, Robert H.. "Sugar: The Bitter Truth." University of California Television. Retrieved from https://www.youtube.com/watch?v=dBnniua6-oM.

Chapter 4

1. Bakris, George L. (March 2013). "High Blood Pressure." *The Merck Manual, Home Health Handbook.* Merck Sharp & Dohme Corp, Merck & Co., Inc. Retrieved from http://www.merckmanuals.com/home/heart_and_blood _vessel _disorders/high_blood_pressure/high_blood_pressure.htm

2. Kumar, Nilay, et al (2015). "A content analysis of smartphone–based applications for hypertension management." *Journal of the American Society of Hypertension* 9.2: 130-136.

3. April 23, 2013). "Anti-Hypertensive Drugs." Baylor Healthcare System. *News-Medical.Net.* Retrieved from http://www.news-medical.net/admin/health/Anti-Hypertensive -Drugs.aspx

4. Neel, Armon B. (February 7, 2013). "Do You Have a Cough That Won't Go Away?" *AARP.org.* Retrieved from http://member.aarp.org/health/drugs-supplements/info-02-2013 /chronic-cough-ace-inhibitors.html

Chapter 5

1. Moss, Michael. *Salt, Sugar, Fat: How the Food Giants Hooked Us.* New York: Random House, 2013.

2. Lepage, Patricia, et al. "A Metagenomic Insight Into Our Gut's Microbiome." *Gut* 62.1 (2013): 146-158.

3. Mayer, Anne-Marie (1997). "Historical changes in the mineral content of fruits and vegetables." *British Food Journal* 99.6: 207-211.

4. Barański, Marcin, et al (2014). "Higher antioxidant and lower cadmium concentrations and lower incidence of pesticide residues in organically grown crops: a systematic literature review and meta-analyses." *British Journal of Nutrition* 112.05: 794-81.

5. Vermeulen, E. G., C. D. Stehouwer, J. W. Twisk, M. Van den Berg, S.C. De Jong, A. J. Mackaay, and J. A. Rauwerda (2000). "Effect of homocysteine-lowering treatment with folic acid plus vitamin B 6 on progression of subclinical atherosclerosis: a randomised, placebo-controlled trial." *The Lancet* 355.9203: 517-522. Retrieved from http://www.ncbi.nlm.nih.gov/pubmed/10683000.

6. Friso, S., V. Lotto, R. Corrocher, and S. W. Choi (2012). "Vitamin b6 and cardiovascular disease in Water Soluble Vitamins." 265-290. Retrieved from http://www.ncbi.nlm.nih.gov/pubmed/22116704.

7. Qin, X., F. Fan, Y. Cui, F. Chen, Y. Chen, X. Cheng, and X. Wang (2014). "Folic acid supplementation with and without vitamin B6 and revascularization risk: A meta-analysis of randomized controlled trials." *Clinical Nutrition* 33.4: 603-612. Retrieved from http://www.ncbi.nlm.nih.gov/pubmed/24461473.

8. Schnyder, G., M. Roffi , Y. Flammer, R. Pin, and O. M. Hess (2002). "Effect of homocysteine-lowering therapy with folic acid, vitamin B12, and vitamin B6 on clinical outcome after percutaneous coronary intervention: the Swiss Heart study: a randomized controlled trial." *Journal of the American Medical Association* 288.8: 973-979. Retrieved from http://www.ncbi.nlm.nih.gov/pubmed/12190367.

9. Yang, H. T., M. Lee, K. S. Hong, B. Ovbiagele, and J. L. Saver (2012). "Efficacy of folic acid supplementation in cardiovascular disease prevention: an updated meta-analysis of randomized controlled trials." *European Journal of Internal Medicine* 23.8: 745-754. Retrieved from http://www.sciencedirect.com/science/article/pii/S0953620512001793.

10. Tian, R., and J. S. Ingwall (2008). "How does folic acid cure heart attacks?." *Circulation* 117.14: 1772-1774. Retrieved from http://circ.ahajournals.org/content/117/14/1772.full.

11. Moens, A. L., H. C. Champion, M. J. Claeys, B. Tavazzi, P. M. Kaminski, M. S. Wolin, and D. A. Kass (2008). "High-dose folic acid pretreatment blunts cardiac dysfunction during ischemia coupled to maintenance of high- energy phosphates and reduces postreperfusion injury." *Circulation* 117.14: 1810-1819. Retrieved from http://www.ncbi.nlm.nih.gov/pubmed/18362233.

12. Pawlak, R. (2015). "Is Vitamin B-12 Deficiency a Risk Factor for Cardiovascular Disease in Vegetarians?" *American Journal of Preventive Medicine* 48.6: e11-e26. Retrieved from http://www.sciencedirect.com/science/ article/pii/S0749379715000732.

13. Yajnik, C. S., H. G. Lubree, N. V. Thuse, L. V. Ramdas, S. S. Deshpande, V. U. Deshpande and R. Efsum (2007). "Oral vitamin B12 supplementation reduces plasma total homocysteine concentration in women in India." *Asia Pacific Journal of Clinical Nutrition* 16.1: 103-9. Retrieved from http://www.ncbi.nlm.nih.gov/pubmed/17215186.

14. El Asmar, M. S., J. J. Naoum, and E. J. Arbid (2014). " Vitamin k dependent proteins and the role of vitamin k2 in the modulation of vascular calcification: a review." *Oman Medical Journal* 29.3: 172. Retrieved from http://www.ncbi.nlm.nih.gov/pubmed/24936265.

15. *Ibid.*

16. Brandenburg, V.M., L. J. Schurgers, N. Kaesler, K. Püsche, R. H. van Gorp, G. Leftheriotis, and T. Krüger (2015). "Prevention of vasculopathy by vitamin K supplementation: Can we turn fiction into fact?" *Atherosclerosis* 240.1: 10-16. Retrieved from http://www.sciencedirect.com/science/article/pii/S0021915015001306.

17. Bolland, M. J., A. Grey, A. Avenell, G. D. Gamble, and I. R. Reid (2011). "Calcium supplements with or without vitamin D and risk of cardiovascular events: reanalysis of the Women's Health Initiative limited access dataset and meta-analysis." *BMJ 342.* Retrieved from http://www.ncbi.nlm.nih.gov/pubmed/21505219.

18. Lundberg, G. D. (November 2014). "Is vitamin K the new vitamin D?" *Medscape Multispecial.* Retrieved from http://www.medscape.com/viewarticle/834763.

19. Glassman, Keri (February 14, 2013). "5 Things You Can Do This Month To Make Your Heart Healthier." *Nutritious Life.com.* Retrieved from http://www.nutritiouslife.com/nlts/5-things-you-can-do-this-month-to-make-your-heart-healthier/.

20. (June 4, 2007). "Omega-3 fatty acids reduce blood pressure: study" Retrieved from http://www.reuters.com/article/us-heart-pressure-omega-idUSN0448551520070604.

21. *Ibid.*

22. Lands, W. E.M. (2005). "Dietary Fat and Health: The Evidence and the Politics of Prevention: Careful Use of Dietary Fats Can Improve Life and Prevent Disease". Annals of the New York Academy of Sciences. 1055: 179–92.

23. Hibbeln, Joseph R; Nieminen, Levi RG; Blasbalg, Tanya L; Riggs, Jessica A; Lands, William EM (2006). "Healthy intakes of n—3 and n—6 fatty acids: estimations considering worldwide diversity". The American Journal of Clinical Nutrition. 83 (6 Suppl): 1483S–1493S.

24. Okuyama, H.; Ichikawa, Y.; Sun, Y.; Hamazaki, T.; Lands, W.E.M. (2006). "ω3 Fatty Acids Effectively Prevent Coronary Heart Disease and Other Late-Onset Diseases – The Excessive Linoleic Acid Syndrome". In Okuyama, H. Prevention of Coronary Heart Disease. World Review of Nutrition and Dietetics. pp. 83–103.

25. Geleijnse, F. J. Kok, and D. E. Grobbee (2003). "Blood pressure response to changes in sodium and potassium intake: a metaregression analysis of randomised trials." *Journal of Human Hypertension* 17:471-480.

26. Walker, W.G., H. Saito, P.K. Whelton, R. P. Russell, and J. S. Herman (1980). "An association between the renin angiotensin system, blood pressure and potassium intake." *Transactions of the American Clinical and Climatological Association* 91: 107-114.

27. *Ibid.*

28. *Ibid.*

29. Kass. L., J Weekes, L Carpenter (March 2012). "Effect of magnesium supplementation on blood pressure: a meta-analysis." *European Journal of Clinical Nutrition.*

30. Cavagnaro, Pablo F., et al (2007). "Effect of cooking on garlic (Allium sativum L.) antiplatelet activity and thiosulfinates content." *Journal of Agricultural and Food Chemistry* 55.4: 1280-1288.

31. Borlinghaus, Jan, et al (2014). "Allicin: chemistry and biological properties." *Molecules* 19.8: 12591-618.

32. Grzybowski, Andrzej, and Krzysztof Pietrzak (2013). "Albert Szent-Györgyi (1893-1986): the scientist who discovered vitamin C." *Clinics in Dermatology* 31.3: 327-331.

33. Prescott, Bonnie. (May 9, 2012). "Falvonoid compound can prevent blood clots." *Harvard Gazette.* Retrieved from http://news.harvard.edu/gazette/story/2012/05/flavonoid -compound-can-prevent-blood-clots/.

34. Choi, Jun-Hui, et al (2015). "Anti-thrombotic effect of rutin isolated from Dendropanax morbifera Leveille." *Journal of Bioscience and Bioengineering* 120.2: 181-186.

35. Yang, Y. C., F. H. Lu, J. S. Wu, et al (July 26, 2004). "The protective effect of habitual tea consumption on hypertension." *Archives of Internal Medicine* 164:1534-1540.

36. *Ibid.*

37. Onakpoya, I., E. Spencer, C. Heneghan, and M. Thompson (2014). "The effect of green tea on blood pressure and lipid profile: A systematic review and meta-analysis of randomized clinical trials." *Nutrition, Metabolism and Cardiovascular Diseases* 24.8: 823-836. Retrieved from http://www.ncbi.nlm.nih.gov/pubmed/24675010.

38. Bogdanski, P., J. Suliburska, M. Szulinska, M. Stepien, D. Pupek-Musialik, and A. Jablecka (2012). "Green tea extract reduces blood pressure, infl ammatory biomarkers, and oxidative stress and improves parameters associated with insulin resistance in obese, hypertensive patients." *Nutrition Research* 32.6: 427. Retrieved from http:// www.ncbi.nlm.nih.gov/pubmed/22749178.

39. Suliburska, J., P. Bogdanski, M. Szulinska, M. Stepien, D. Pupek-Musialik, and A. Jablecka (2012). " Effects of green tea supplementation on elements, total antioxidants, lipids, and glucose values in the serum of obese patients." *Biological Trace Element Research* 149.3: 315-322. Retrieved from http://www.ncbi.nlm.nih.gov/pubmed/22581111.

40. "Diseases and Conditions: Metabolic Syndrome." *Mayo Foundation for Medical Education and Research.* Retrieved from http://www.mayoclinic.org/diseases-conditions/metabolic -syndrome/multimedia/apple-and-pear-body- shapes/img -20006114.

41. Li, Gi., Y. Zhang, L. Thabane, L. Mbuagbaw, A. Liu, M. A. Levine, and A. Holbrook (2015). "Effect of green tea supplementation on blood pressure among overweight and obese adults: a systematic review and meta-analysis." *Journal of Hypertension* 33.2:243-254. Retrieved from http://www.ncbi.nlm.nih.gov/pubmed/25479028.

42. Diepvens, Kristel, Klaas R. Westerterp, and Margriet S. Westerterp-Plantenga (2007). "Obesity and thermogenesis related to the consumption of caffeine, ephedrine, capsaicin, and green tea." *American Journal of Physiology-Regulatory, Integrative and Comparative Physiology* 292.1: R77-R85.

43. Bone, Kerry, and Simon Mills (January 8, 2013). "Principles and Practice of Phytotherapy." *Modern Herbal Medicine 2nd edition*.

44. Meschino, James, DC, MS, ND, ROHP, RAP (March 18, 2013.) "Hawthorn, The Three- In-One Natural Remedy For High Blood Pressure." *Meschino Health.com*. Retrieved from http://www.meschinohealth.com/ArticleDirectory/Hawthorn_Natural_Blood_Pressure_Remedy.

45. Heber. D., N. P. Seeram, H. Wyatt, S. M. Henning, Y. Zhang, L. G. Ogden, and J. O. Hill (2007). "Safety and antioxidant activity of a pomegranate ellagitannin-enriched polyphenol dietary supplement in overweight individuals with increased waist size." *Journal of Agricultural and Food Chemistry* 55.24: 10050-10054. Retrieved from http://www.ncbi.nlm.nih.gov/pubmed/17966977

46. Gil. M. I., F. A. Tomás-Barberán, B. Hess-Pierce, D. M. Holcroft, and A. A. Kade (2000). "Antioxidant activity of pomegranate juice and its relationship with phenolic composition and processing." *Journal of Agricultural and Food Chemistry* 48.10: 4581-4589.

47. Aviram, M., and L. Dornfeld (2001). "Pomegranate juice consumption inhibits serum angiotensin converting enzyme activity and reduces systolic blood pressure." *Atherosclerosis* 158.1: 195-198. Retrieved from http://www.ncbi.nlm. nih.gov/pubmed/11500191.

48. Zarfeshany, A., S. Asgary, and S. H. Javanmard (2014). " Potent health effects of pomegranate." *Advanced Biomedical Research*. Retrieved from http://www.ncbi.nlm.nih.gov/pubmed/24800189.

49. "Heart Disease and C-Reactive Protein (CRP) Testing." *Heart Disease Health Center.* Retrieved from http://www.webmd.com/heart-disease/guide/heart-disease-c-reactive-protein-crp-testing.

50. Antony, B., M. Benny, and T.N.B. Kaimal (2008). " A Pilot clinical study to evaluate the effect of Emblica officinalis extract on markers of systemic inflammation and dyslipidemia." *Indian Journal of Clinical Biochemistry* 23.4:378-381. Retrieved from http://www.ncbi.nlm.nih.gov/ pubmed/23105791.

51. Pradyumna, T., Rao, T. Okamoto, N. Akita, T. Hayashi, N. Kato-Yasuda, and K. Suzuki (2013). "Amlamax™ (Emblica officinalis) extract inhibits lipopolysaccharide-induced procoagulant and pro-inflammatory factors in cultured vascular endothelial cells." *British Journal of Nutrition* 110.12: 2201-2206. Retrieved from http://www.ncbi.nlm.nih.gov/pubmed/23742702.

52. Antony, B., B. Merina, and V. Sheeba (2008). "Amlamax™ in the Management of Dyslipidemia in Humans." Indian journal of pharmaceutical sciences, 70.4: 504. Retrieved from http://www.ncbi.nlm.nih.gov/pubmed/20046781.

53. Akhtar, M. S., A. Ramzan, A. Ali, and M. Ahmad, M. (2011). " Effect of Amla fruit (Emblica officinalis Gaertn.) on blood glucose and lipid profile of normal subjects and type 2 diabetic patients." *International Journal of Food Sciences and Nutrition* 62.6: 609-616. Retrieved from http://www.ncbi.nlm.nih.gov/pubmed/21495900.

54. Bhatt, J., and K. G. Hemavathi (2012). " Acomparative clinical study of hypolipidemic efficacy of Amla (Emblica officinalis) with 3-hydroxy-3-methylglutaryl-coenzyme-A reductase inhibitor simvastatin." *Indian Journal of Pharmacology* 44.2: 238. Retrieved from http://www.ncbi.nlm.nih.gov/pubmed/22529483.

55. Aubrey, Allison (August 28, 2008). "To Lower Blood Pressure, Open Up and Say 'Om.'" *NPR.org.* Retrieved from http://www.npr.org/2008/08/21/93796200/to-lower-blood-pressure-open-up-and-say-om.

Bibliography

- Davis, William (March 2010). "Reduce Blood Pressure—Naturally-What Americans Can Learn from Traditional Cultures about Managing Hypertension." *Life Extension Magazine.*

- Bertrand, Jessica (October 23, 2012). "Flavonoids and Cardiovascular Health." *AH-A, Agri-Food For Healthy Aging.* Retrieved from http://aha.the-ria.ca/blog/?p=1250.

- Mayer, Anne-Marie. "Historical changes in the mineral content of fruits and vegetables." British Food Journal 99.6 (1997): 207-211.

- Barański, Marcin, et al. "Higher antioxidant and lower cadmium concentrations and lower incidence of pesticide residues in organically grown crops: a systematic literature review and meta-analyses." British Journal of Nutrition 112.05 (2014): 794-811.

- Hobbs, Christopher (March 18, 2013). "The Heart Herbs: Hawthorn and Garlic." *Healthy.net.* Retrieved from http://www.healthy.net/scr/article.aspx?Id=899"/scr/article.aspx?Id=899.

- Paknikar, Simi (January 10, 2012). "Garlic Lowers Blood Pressure in Hypertensive Patients." *MedIndia.* Health In Focus. Retrieved from http://www.medindia.net/news/healthinfocus/Garlic-Lowers -Blood-Pressure-in-Hypertensive-Patients-95906-1.htm.

- (March 6, 2013). "Dietary Supplement Fact Sheet: Calcium." *Natural Institutes of Health.* Retrieved from http:// ods.od.nih.gov/factsheets/Calcium-HealthProfessional/.

- (October 12, 2012). "Dietary Supplement Fact Sheet: Selenium." Office of Dietary Supplements. *National Institute of Health.* Retrieved from http://ods.od.nih.gov/factsheets/Selenium-HealthProfessional/ http://ods.od.nih.gov/ factsheets/Selenium-HealthProfessional/#h6/.

- Carla (January 15, 2010). "Health Benefits of Mustard Seeds." *Herbal Remedies and Natural Health.* Retrieved from http://guide2herbalremedies.com/health-benefits-mustard-seeds/.

- *The World's Healthiest Foods.* The George Mateljan Foundation. Retrieved from http://www.whfoods.com/genpage.php?tname=foodspice&dbid=106.

- Brody, Jane E. (February 19, 1997). "Hopes Rising for Selenium." *New York Times.* Retrieved from http://www. nytimes.com/1997/02/19/us/hopes-rising-for-selenium.html.

- Sparacino-Watkins, Courtney E., Yen-Chun Lai, and Mark T. Gladwin (2012). "Nitrate-nitrite-nitric oxide pathway in pulmonary arterial hypertension therapeutics." 112.

- Gokce, N. (October 2004). "L-Arginine and hypertension." *Journal of Nutrition* 134.10: 2807S–2811S. Retrieved from http://www.ncbi.nlm.nih.gov/pubmed/1546579015465790.

- Roberts, Christine (January 05, 2011). "Pass the mustard and those health benefits please." *NaturalNews.com.* Retrieved from http://www.naturalnews.com/030916_mustard_health_food.html.

- Carlström, M., et al. (2011). "Dietary nitrate attenuates oxidative stress, prevents cardiac and renal injuries, and reduces blood pressure in salt-induced hypertension." *Cardiovascular Research* 89.3: 574.

- Penelope, Andrew J. (August 15, 1999). "Enzymatic function of nitric oxide synthases". *Oxford Journal.* Retrieved from http://cardiovascres.oxfordjournals.org/content/43/3/521.

- Zeratsky, Katherine (March 5, 2013). "What's the difference between sea salt and table salt?" *Mayo Foundation for Medical Education and Research.* Retrieved from http://www.mayoclinic.com/health/sea-salt/AN01142.

- Shannon (February 25, 2010). *Simple Living Media.* Retrieved from Simplebites.net.

- Gittleman, Anne Louise (March 5, 2013). "Understanding Salt and Sodium."

- (March 27, 2012). "Hot pepper compound could help hearts." American Chemical Society. *Science Daily.*

- (August 2010). "Activation of TRPV1 by Dietary Capsaicin Improves Endothelium-Dependent Vasorelaxation and Prevents Hypertension." *Cell Symposia* 12.2: 130–141. Retrieved from http://dx.doi.org/10.1016/cmet.2010.05.015.

- Wong, Cathy (Updated September 24, 2012). "Alternative Medicine." *About.com.* Retrieved from http://dx.doi.org/10.3949/ccjm.77a.09078"doi.org/10.3949/ccjm.77a.09078.

- (December 2005). "Essential fatty acids." *Linus Pauling Institute.* Retrieved from http://lpi.oregonstate.edu/infocenter/othernuts/omega3fa/index.html#food_source.

- Heyes, J.D. (December 30, 2012). "Lower Your Blood Pressure Significantly with Omega-3 Fatty Acids." *Natural News Network.* Retrieved from. http://www.naturalnews.com/038507_blood_pressure_omega-3_fatty_acids.html.

- Wong, Cathy (September 24, 2012). "Natural Remedies for High Blood Pressure." *About.com.* Retrieved from http://altmedicine.about.com/cs/herbsvitaminsek/a/Hypertension.htm.

- Hobbs, Christopher. "The Heart Herbs: Hawthorn and Garlic." *Healthy.net.* Retrieved from http://www.healthy.net/scr/article.aspx?Id=899.

- Mullins, Brittany (February 20, 2012). "Health Benefits of Apple Cider Vinegar (ACV)." Retrieved from http://www.eatingbirdfood.com/2012/02/health-benefits-of-apple-cider-vinegar-acv/.

- Mathias, Kevin (January 2, 2013.). "Health Benefi ts of Apple Cider Vinegar." *Buzzle.com.* Retrieved www. buzzle.com/articles/health-benefi ts-apple-cider-vinegar.html.

- Wendler, Jim (December 19, 2011). "Blood Pressure Remedy-Apple Cider Vinegar." Retrieved from http://www.jimwendler.com/2011/12/blood-pressure-remedy-apple-cider-vinegar/.

The Blood Pressure Solution

- Lori, L. (November 15, 2009). "Apple Cider Vinegar for High Blood Pressure Treatment- Part 2 in a series about Apple Cider Vinegar." *Natural Healing Remedies.* Retrieved from. http://naturalhealingremedies.org/index.php/2009/11/apple-cider-vinegar-for-high-blood-pressure-treatment/.

- Smith, Jack L., and Sareen S. Gropper (February 10, 2010). *Advanced Nutrition and Human Metabolism,* 5th Edition. Cengage Learning.

- Weil, Andrew (August 30, 2012.). "High Blood Pressure, Hypertension. Condition Care Guide." *Weil Lifestyle.* Retrieved from http://www.drweil.com/drw/u/ART00686/high-blood-pressure-treatment.

- Phillip, John (September 12, 2012.) "Vitamin C lowers blood pressure, improves vascular function to lower heart attack and stroke risk." *NaturalNews.com.* Retrieved from http://www.naturalnews.com/037163_ vitamin_c_blood_pressure_heart_attack_risk.html.

- (April 4, 2012). "Effects of vitamin C supplementation on blood pressure: a meta-analysis of randomized controlled trials." *American Cancer Society.* Retrieved from http://ajcn.nutrition.org/content/95/5/1079.

- Boshtam, M., M. Rafiei, K. Sadeghi, and N. Sarraf-Zadegan (October 2002). "Vitamin E can reduce blood pressure in mild hypertensives." *National Center for Biotechnology Information, U.S. National Library of Medicine.* Retrieved from. http://www.ncbi.nlm.nih.gov/pubmed/12463106.

- (October 11, 2011). "Dietary Supplement Fact Sheet: Vitamin E." *NIH Office of Dietary Supplements.* Retrieved from. http://ods.od.nih.gov/factsheets/VitaminE-QuickFacts/?print=1.

- "Facts about Vitamin E." *Healing Edgs Sciences, Inc.* Retrieved from http://www.healingedge.net/store/article_vitamin_e.html.

- Forman, John P., et al. (2007). "Plasma 25-hydroxyvitamin D levels and risk of incident hypertension." *Hypertension* 49.5:1063-1069.

- Price, Paul A., Jessica R. Buckley, and Matthew K. Williamson (2001). "The amino bisphosphonate ibandronate prevents vitamin D toxicity and inhibits vitamin D-induced calcification of arteries, cartilage, lungs and kidneys in rats." *The Journal of Nutrition* 131.11: 2910-2915.

- (25 Apr. 2012) "Vitamin D supplements can reduce blood pressure in patients with hypertension." *Science Daily.* Retrieved from http://dx.doi.org/10.1007/s12170-011-0186-0

- Mercola, Joseph (October 10, 2009). "How Much Vitamin D Do You Really Need to Take?" *Natural Health Website.* Retrieved from http://articles.mercola.com/sites/articles/archive/2009/10/10/Vitamin-D-Experts-Reveal-the-Truth.aspx.

- Bagchia, D., Chandan K Senb, Sidhartha D Rayc, Dipak K Dasd, Manashi Bagchia, Harry G Preusse, and Joe A Vinsonf (March 2003). "Molecular mechanisms of cardioprotection by a novel grape seed proanthocyanidin extract". *ScienceDirect.* Retrieved from http://dx.doi.org/10.1016/S0027-5107(02)00324-X.

- Feringa, H.H. MD, PhD; Dayne A. Laskey, PharmD; Justine E. Dickson, PharmD; and Craig I. Coleman (August 2011). "The Effect of Grape Seed Extract on Cardiovascular Risk." *Journal of American Dietetic Association.* Retrieved from http://dx.doi.org/10.1016/j.jada.2011.05.015.

- Richards, Byron J. "Grape Seed Extract Lowers Blood Pressure." *WellnessResources.com.*

- (June 9, 2011). "Water: How much should you drink every day?" *Mayo Foundation for Medical Education and Research.* Retrieved from. http://www.mayoclinic.com/health/AboutThisSite/AM00057.

- (January 2005) "Insufficient Sleep Associated With Overweight And Obesity." *Journal Of The American Medical Association.*

- "Increased Fructose Associates with Elevated Blood Pressure" *PubMed.gov.* Retrieved from http://www.ncbi.nlm.nih.gov/pubmed/20595676.

- Buchanan, Duncan S., Stewart Ollis, John D. Young, Non E. Thomas, Stephen-Mark Cooper, Tom Tong, Jinlei Nie, Robert M. Malina, and S. Julien (April 4, 2011). "The effects of time and intensity of exercise on novel and established markers of CVD in adolescent youth." *Wiley Library Online.* Retrieved from http://dx.doi.org/10.1002/ajhb.21166.

- Dusek, Jeffery A., et al (2008). "Stress management versus lifestyle modifi cation on systolic hypertension and medication elimination: a randomized trial." *The Journal of Alternative and Complementary Medicine* 14.2: 138.

- Epel, Elissa S., et al (2012). "Wandering minds and aging cells." Clinical Psychological Science.

- Anderson, James W., Chunxu Liu, and Richard J. Kryscio (September 7, 2007). "Blood Pressure Response to Transcendental Meditation: A Meta-analysis." *American Journal of Hypertension*. Retrieved from http://doi.org/10.1038/ajh.2007.65.

- Wahbeh, Helané ND; Siegward-M Elsas, MD; and Barry S. Oken, MD (June 10, 2008). "Mind Body Interventions."

- *American Academy of Neurology.* Retrieved from http://dx.doi.org/10.1212/01.wnl.0000314667.16386.5e.

- "Stress and high blood pressure: What's the Connection?" *Mayo Foundation for Medical Education and Research.* Retrieved from http://www.mayoclinic.com/health/stress-and-high-blood -pressure/HI00092.

- Kiks. "Basic Meditation Techniques." ProjectMeditation.org. Retrieved from http://www.project-meditation.org/a_mt4/basic _meditation_techniques.html.

- Jones, Mary. "Guided Meditation." *Project-Meditation.org.* Retrieved from http://www.project-meditation.org/mt/guided _meditation.html.

- Kundan, Pandey. "Deep Breathing Exercises to Lower Blood Pressure." *Buzzle.com.*

- "The Complete Guide to Binaural Beats." *Binauralbrains.com.*

- "Acupuncture." *Mayo Foundation for Medical Education and Research.* Retrieved from http://www.mayoclinic.com/health/acupuncture/MY00946.

- Springer, Robin (September 11, 2012). "Can Acupuncture Help Lower High Blood Pressure?" *Essential Wellness.* Retrieved from http://essentialwellnesssf.com/2012/09/can-acupuncture-help-lower-high-blood-pressure/.

- (February 6, 2013). "Acupuncture to lower blood Pressure." *Onlymyhealth.com.*

- (October, 2004). "Study: Daily Tea Consumption Reduces Risk of Hypertension." *Acupuncture Today* 5.10. Retrieved from http://healthsolutionssource.com/StudyDailyTeaConsumption.pdf.

- Salamon, Maureen (September 21, 2012). "Poor Sleep May Make High Blood Pressure Worse." *U.S. News & World Report.*

- (December 10, 2012). "Sleeping Longer At Night Could Improve Blood Pressure Levels: Study." *HuffingtonPost.com.* Retrieved from http://www.huffingtonpost.com/2012/12/10/sleep-blood-pressure-duratiobedtime-hypertension_n_2238135.html.

- "Sleep Tips: 7 steps to better sleep." *Mayo Foundation for Medical Education and Research.* Retrieved from, http://www.mayoclinic.com/health/sleep/HQ01387.

- (March 23, 2009). "Autogenic Training and Biofeedback." *Natural Health.com.* Retrieved from http://natural-health.most-effective-solution.com/2009/03/autogenic-training-and-biofeedback/.

- "Diseases and Conditions: Metabolic Syndrome." *Mayo Foundation for Medical Education and Research.* Retrieved from http://www.mayoclinic.org/diseases-conditions/metabolic-syndrome/multimedia/apple-and-pear-body-shapes/img-20006114.

- Kaufmann, Lauren (June 22, 2012). "Eight Natural Ways To Lower Blood Pressure." *Health Fair.* Retrieved from http://www.healthfair.com/eight-natural-ways-lower-blood-pressure/.

- (March 2012). "Hypertension/High Blood Pressure." *Web MD.*

- University of Maryland Medical Center (March 6, 2013). "Lifestyle changed needed to control high blood pressure."

- Wong, Cathy (September 2013). "Herbs, Vitamins, Hypertension." *About.com.* Retrieved from http://altmedicine.about.com/cs/herbsvitaminsek/a/Hypertension.htm.

- (March 2013). "Top 10 Vegetables Highest in Potassium." *Healthaliciousness.com.*

- Geboy, Alexander G. , Dawn M. Filmyer, and Richard C. Josiassen (2012). "Motor Deficits Associated With Mild, Chronic Hyponatremia: A Factor Analytic Study." *Journal of Motor Behavior* 44.4: 255-259.

- Zamanian, Roham T., et al. (2009). "Insulin resistance in pulmonary arterial hypertension." *European Respiratory Journal* 33.2: 318-324.

- (April 12, 2013). "Most Americans Consume Too Much Sodium." *Centers for Disease Control and Prevention.* Retrieved from http://www.cdc.gov/bloodpressure/sodium.htm.

- Suz (May 2, 2012). "The DASH Diet." *The Paleo Network.* Retrieved from http://paleo.com.au/2012/05/dash-diet/.

- Cordain, Loren, Janette Brand Miller, S Boyd Eaton, Neil Mann, Susanne HA Holt, and John D Speth (March 2000). "Plant-animal subsistence ratios and macronutrient energy estimations in worldwide hunter-gatherer diets". *The American Journal of Clinical Nutrition* 71.3: 682-692. Retrieved from http://ajcn.nutrition.org/search?author1=Loren+Cordain&sortspec=date&submit=Submit.

Trademarks

Images used under license from Shutterstock.com.

Viagra® is a registered trademark of Pfizer Inc.

My Fitness Pal® is a registered trademark of Under Armour, Inc.

LoseIt!® is a registered trademark of FitNow, Inc.